THE METHODOLOGY OF DISCOURSE ANALYSIS

T5-DGK-569

Penny Powers

NLN
PRESS

THE METHODOLOGY OF DISCOURSE ANALYSIS

Penny Powers, Ph.D., R.N.
South Dakota State University
College of Nursing

JONES AND BARTLETT PUBLISHERS
Sudbury, Massachusetts
BOSTON   TORONTO   LONDON   SINGAPORE

National League for Nursing

World Headquarters
Jones and Bartlett Publishers
40 Tall Pine Drive
Sudbury, MA 01776
978-443-5000
www.jbpub.com
info@jbpub.com

Jones and Bartlett Publishers Canada
2406 Nikanna Road
Mississauga, ON L5C 2W6
CANADA

Jones and Bartlett Publishers International
Barb House, Barb Mews
London W6 7PA
UK

Library of Congress Cataloging-in-Publication Data

Powers, Penny, 1948-
   The methodology of discourse analysis / Penny Powers.
       p. cm.
   Includes bibliographical references and index.
   ISBN 0-7637-1804-1 (alk. paper)
   1. Discourse analysis. 2. Nursing—Research. I. Title.

   RT81.5 .P694 2001
   610.73'07'2—dc21

                                                            2001028058

Production Credits
Acquisitions Editor: Penny M. Glynn
Associate Editor: Christine Tridente
Production Editor: AnnMarie Lemoine
Editorial Assistant: Thomas Prindle
Manufacturing Buyer: Amy Duddridge
Cover Design: AnnMarie Lemoine
Design and Composition: Carlisle Communications, Ltd.
Printing and Binding: Malloy Lithographing

Printed in the United States of America
05 04 03 02 01   10 9 8 7 6 5 4 3 2 1

PREFACE

The methodology of discourse analysis is more familiar to researchers in Western Europe than it is to readers in the United States. Although there have been some excellent analyses written of discourses in the United States, the method remains largely unknown, and isolated researchers in sociology, dentistry, linguistics, psychology, social work, anthropology, and nursing are not sharing methodological considerations with each other. This volume intends to remedy the situation by placing discourse analysis squarely within the interpretive paradigm among other, more seasoned members and by making it accessible to all.

The intended audience for this book consists of faculty and graduate students interested in qualitative research methods in general and oppression and emancipation in particular. In our post-colonial world, interest in qualitative research methods that are openly gendered moral analyses of power relations is increasing. Qualitative researchers have faced (and have overcome) several crises (Denzin, 1997). These crises, precipitated for the most part by the postmodern turn, have challenged perspectives in all of the social sciences.

To be sure, there are differences of opinion among researchers using ethnography, feminism, critical hermeneutics, queer theory, performance text, participatory action research, and others. What is becoming clear, however, is that considerable agreement exists with regard to some very key issues. First and foremost is the agreement that our understanding of the "real world" is a social construction. The tension between this social construction and a researcher's interpretation of it (another social construction) gives rise to some very fruitful discussions regarding the role of researcher as social agent.

Secondly, the goal of interpretive research is radical political action. No one apologizes for this anymore. Interpretive claims produced by postpositivist qualitative methods represent agendas and values as clearly as the claims made by empirical research. The difference is that in the qualitative claims, the values and agendas are stated up front, rather than as an interpretation.

What you will find in this book may seem like a "cookbook" approach. I assure you that this suggested approach is just that—*suggested*. Hybrid approaches to qualitative research methods are being used (Denzin & Lincoln,

2000), but it is important to be aware of the assumptions of the method chosen. Researchers cannot use multiple regression if the data do not conform to the assumptions of the method. Similarly, there are incommensurable assumptions behind the methods of phenomenology and discourse analysis.

Chapter 1 presents the theoretical, philosophical, and conceptual underpinnings of the method of discourse analysis. Chapter 2 presents the feminist contribution to discourse analysis, and Chapter 3 details the suggested steps in the method. Chapter 4 presents an example of a discourse analysis in nursing: a discourse analysis of nursing diagnosis.

The choice of example analysis for the book, the discourse analysis of nursing diagnosis, may confuse readers whose discipline is not nursing. However, as a controversial concept, it is an excellent candidate for discourse analysis and can serve as an example of what it looks and sounds like when the suggested method in this book is followed.

As a White, middle-aged female and academic Canadian-American nurse, I am aware of my considerable privilege in life. This place, however, gives me a position from which to speak that is denied to others. I consider this a useful tool and intend to make use of it. This book is an effort in the direction of providing a tool for people who wish to analyze discourses in their own discipline, neighborhood, or household.

Penny Powers, Ph.D., R.N.
Brookings, South Dakota, January 18, 2001

REFERENCES

Denzin, N. K. (1997). *Interpretive ethnography: Ethnographic practices for the 21st century.* Thousand Oaks, CA: Sage.

Denzin, N. K., & Lincoln, Y. S. (2000). *Handbook of qualitative research* (2nd ed.). Thousand Oaks, CA: Sage.

CONTENTS

CHAPTER 1

THE THEORETICAL FOUNDATIONS OF DISCLOSURE ANALYSIS

INTRODUCTION

Discourse analysis is a relatively recent approach to the examination of systematic bodies of knowledge in the tradition of critical social theory and poststructural, postmodern feminism (Gavey, 1997; Gray, 1999; Hinshaw, Feetham, & Shaver, 1999; McNay, 1992). Discourse analysis may be performed in different ways, but all of the procedural variations share common goals and assumptions. The application to diverse disciplines has so far prevented a completely coherent perspective (Cheek & Rudge, 1994). Discourse analysis differs from other traditions such as semiotics and ethnomethodology in that discourse analysis emphasizes the power inherent in social relations (Lupton, 1992).

One of the possible methodologies for discourse analysis is derived from the works of Michel Foucault, French philosopher and historian. This book describes the theoretical foundations of discourse analysis, discusses the methodology, describes the production of a discourse analysis, and gives one example of a completed discourse analysis from the discipline of nursing. Discourse analysis deserves consideration as an interpretive methodology for nursing inquiry (Cheek & Rudge, 1994).

Discourse has been defined as "a group of ideas or patterned way of thinking which can be identified in textual and verbal communications, and can also be located in wider social structures" (Lupton, 1992, p. 145). The methodology of discourse analysis provides insight into the functioning of bodies of knowledge in their specific situated context (Cheek, 1997). Discourse analysis generates interpretive claims with regard to the effects of a discourse on the oppression and empowerment of groups of people in a specific context without claims of generalizability.

This chapter will situate discourse analysis among some other traditions of research and social critique so that the reader can understand where it came from and what it purports to do. Chapter 2 describes the feminist contribution to the theoretical approach and methodology of discourse analysis. Chapter 3 presents a possible method of performing a discourse analysis, and chapter 4 presents an example of a completed discourse analysis: an analysis of the discourse of nursing diagnosis.

Discourse analysis is based on several historical developments in the philosophy of science, social theory, and literary critique. As an approach to analyzing systematic bodies of knowledge (discourses), discourse analysis participates in several traditions of western thought. These traditions and the influence they have had on the development of discourse analysis will be described. The major theoretical influences on the method of discourse analysis are critical social theory, the work of Michel Foucault, antifoundationalism, postmodernism, and feminism. Each of these influences will be discussed, and the relevance for discourse analysis will be demonstrated.

CRITICAL SOCIAL THEORY

The tradition of critical social theory has roots in Marxist thought and the literary traditions of critique and literary criticism (DeMarco, Cambell, & Wuest, 1993). Critical social theory has been suggested as an appropriate and useful approach for nursing inquiry (Allen, 1985; Dzurec, 1989; Doering, 1992; Hedin, 1986; Thompson, 1985; Thompson, 1987).

What we now call critical social theory arose from the Marxist studies of the Institute of Social Research, which was established in Frankfurt in 1923 and is now called the Frankfurt School (Held, 1980). The work of authors associated with this institute does not form a unified body of work, because there are major differences between the primary authors: Horkheimer, Adorno, Marcuse, Lowenthal, and Pollock. These differences do not, however, preclude us from stating, in some instances, the "position" of critical theorists generally. For a more complete description of critical theory see *Introduction to Critical Theory* by Held (1980). Presently, the name most often associated with critical social theory is Jurgen Habermas, who became an assistant to Adorno in the 1960s and is still extremely influential, albeit more in Europe than in Anglo-American social theory (Held, 1980).

A critical social theory can be defined as a critique of historically based social and political institutions that oppress people, while at the same time having a situated practical intent to decrease such oppression (Leonard, 1990). The practical intent of a critical social theory is intended to provide people with the tools to change oppressive situations, whether it is perceived by or hidden from them. According to Lenoarda critical theory without the practical dimension is therefore called "bankrupt on its own terms" (1990, p. 3).

A critical social theory describes how groups exist in relation to the historically based dominant ideologies that structure their experience. The specific process advocated by critical theory is the bringing about of self-liberating practices among people using descriptions of oppressive conditions. It is not clear exactly how these self-liberating practices are to be brought about, but it is clear that the practices must not be forced upon people by researchers or by anyone else.

Using the notions of ideology and false consciousness, critical theory seeks to identify ways in which social phenomena might be otherwise less oppressive, looking for alternate possibilities inherent in present oppressive circumstances. The ultimate goal of a critical theory is the emancipation of human beings as a consequence of becoming aware of an alternate interpretation, which includes a different and better future. The key notions of ideology and false consciousness will now be addressed in order to understand how the approach of critical social theory to these concepts has influenced discourse analysis.

IDEOLOGY AND FALSE CONSCIOUSNESS

Althusser defines ideology as a "representation of the imaginary relationship of individuals to their real conditions of existence" (1971, p. 162). Althusser argues that ideology is a process that obscures the fact that concealed values are operating in a systematic manner to oppress people. This is to say that ideology is an interpretation of a social relationship; the interpretation (or representation) creates social meaning and has social consequences.

Marxist theory, for example, presents a representation (or interpretation) of the relationship between people and their conditions of existence under the economic system of capitalism. In other words, Marxism presents descriptions of ideologies among the owning class that have the effect of oppressing people in the working class. The representations presented by Marxist theory describe how people (in this case, the working class) are oppressed by the operation of concealed values among the owning class.

Ideology also can be described as the existence and functioning of an oppressive interpretation (or representation, in Althusser's terms) that is hidden to the actors yet is one that they would recognize were it presented to them. Habermas (1971), for example, argued for the existence of ideologies other than capitalism in our advanced industrialized society that function unconsciously as a tool of domination, preventing individuals from perceiving that they are the victims of exploitation in increasing areas of their lives. However, when presented with this representation, critical theorists make the claim that people can recognize the representation and the oppressive consequences of the ideology and make sense of it in their social reality.

According to Marxist theory, the ideology of capitalism produces a false consciousness in the working class: an illusion that the work of individuals results in personal gain. Marxist theory provides the representation (or interpretation) to the working class that their work functions instead only to reproduce the conditions (and relations) of production for benefit, not to themselves, but to the owning class. Marxism therefore claims to describe this oppressive ideology in a way that people can recognize in their lives.

Marxist theory uses the term *false consciousness* because Marxism assumes the existence of a *true* consciousness in which the relations of domination are *revealed*. Marxist theory therefore denies the validity of other possible representations (or interpretations) of the conditions of existence among people under capitalism.

The authors of the Frankfurt School, on the other hand, argued that it is not necessary to assume that there exists an absolutely true version of the *real* interpretation or conditions of existence to which to appeal in the process of determining that deception is happening. It is not necessary to assume that there is some deeply hidden true meaning or interpretation within a discourse that is the cause of a false consciousness (Dreyfus & Rabinow, 1983). Instead, it is argued that people may be deluded by one interpretation of reality, only to be convinced of their delusion by another interpretation that seems to be preferable and/or more explanatory to them in that context. The interpretation may not be any more *true* in some objective sense but may indeed be more *preferable* to people in some situated context and at some point in time. Furthermore, there may be many such competing consciousnesses. Traditions of inquiry such as discourse analysis, feminism, interpretive ethnography, and critical hermeneutics all share this view of preferable explanations with the critical social theorists (Denzin, 1997).

FOUNDATIONALISM AND ITS CRITIQUE BY CRITICAL SOCIAL THEORY

Foundationalism will be discussed in order to demonstrate that the methodology of discourse analysis is antifoundational because it participates in and extends the critique of foundationalism by critical social theory. This discussion will help to explain how the power perspective of a discourse analysis approaches the problems of its own position within the power relations it describes and the problems involved in making recommendations for action called for by Leonard's definition of a critical theory.

The word *foundationalism* describes some of the underlying assumptions of the empirical analytic tradition of scientific inquiry. *Empirical analytic* is to be distinguished from the term *empirical*, which means utilizing empirical or observable evidence as data (Lowenberg, 1993). The empirical analytic tradition is a more narrow approach to the description of an assumed preexisting reality through sense data.

The so-called *natural sciences* are the most commonly cited examples of the empirical analytic tradition and are examples of what is labeled *foundationalism* in contemporary philosophical writings. The natural sciences include physics, biology, and chemistry, and the methods of empirical analytic science were originally designed for, and explicitly aimed toward, technical exploitation and control of natural phenomena (Held, 1980; Kusch, 1991).

Among the critical theorists, Habermas observed that human beings have become both the subjects and the objects of these control strategies that had originally been designed for nature (Kusch, 1991). Habermas (1971) argued that the functioning of science, technology, industry, and administration are intimately connected. These ideologies have produced a continually escalating level of technical control over nature and people in the name of the assumed value-free goals of predictability and efficiency. The critique provided by critical social theorists addressed the foundational assumptions of the empirical analytic tradition of science as described by the empirical school of philosophical thought called *logical positivism*.

Logical positivism is the name given to the philosophical and scientific positions of the Vienna Circle. This group of mathematicians and philosophers began meeting informally in 1907 and continued publishing until the mid-1930s (Passmore, 1967). They attempted to set scientific standards for all significant truth statements in science and assumed that the essence of the concept of scientific knowledge itself was understood (Mish'alani, 1988).

There are four key assumptions in the foundational approach of logical positivism regarding the relationship of truth statements in empirical analytic science to the existence of an objective preexisting uninterpreted reality. These four assumptions are crucial to understanding the critique of foundationalism by critical social theory and by the approach of discourse analysis.

The first assumption is the existence of a *foundation* of uninterpreted or preinterpreted facts in an objectively real world that are available to people through sense perception. Second, it is assumed that direct correspondence between our sense perceptions and these absolutely true (and accessible) facts exists. The third assumption is that fact and value are separate notions independent of one another and that empirical analytic science can deal only with facts without dealing with values at the same time. Fourth, the process of empirical analytic science, dealing only with the true facts of a situation, can therefore discern the philosophical essence of concepts and their relationships, such as the causal relationship (Held, 1980).

On the basis of these foundational assumptions, logical positivism, as described by the Vienna Circle, claimed complete value-freedom for the empirical analytic tradition, also called the scientific method. These assumptions construct a position from which to provide value-free critique of other, competing views. Logical positivism assumes the existence of a transcendental independent basis for the evaluation of competing claims.

Assuming the existence of "bare facts" also allows an independent basis to which to appeal in distinguishing between theoretical and empirical claims. From such a value-free perspective, any research tradition that does not base claims on these "bare facts" can be rejected as illegitimate or irrational.

On the basis of these foundational assumptions, logical positivism claimed that human rationality is therefore limited to the empirical analytic scientific view and denied to all other discourses such as ethics and aesthetics. Science, in this view, is therefore the only mode in which reality can be rationally presented (Held, 1980). It follows that philosophy and ethics have no basis to critique scientific claims because these disciplines admit value judgments, whereas empirical analytic science does not.

It should be noted in this context that some critical theorists reject the separation of fact and value and reject the value-neutrality of the empirical analytic tradition without rejecting the existence of "bare facts" (for example, see Althusser, 1971). In general, however, the critical theorists rejected the claims of foundationalism as described by the logical positivists of the Vienna Circle.

Others applied the foundational assumptions described by logical positivism to the human sciences or social sciences. It was argued that these disciplines could be viewed as evolving toward true scientific status on the model of the natural sciences. Critical theorists and others argued against the assumptions of logical positivism and the extension of these assumptions to the social sciences. Foucault, for example, "was critical of the human sciences as a dubious and dangerous attempt to model a science of human beings on the natural sciences" (Dreyfus, 1987, p. 311).

The authors of the Frankfurt School demonstrated convincingly that foundational claims to true knowledge were not value-free but were clearly tied to certain social projects, values, interests, genders, races, classes, and agendas. They argued that western science had become socially engaged and politically powerful despite (or possibly because of) the claim to value-freedom (Seidman & Wagner, 1992). The critical theorists were indeed skeptical of the existence of any facts purported to lack value and ideological components (Street, 1992).

The critical theorists of the Frankfurt School argued that in the name of the foundational assumption of the value-freedom of science, one certain set of unacknowledged, unstated, and unexamined values had achieved precedence above all others without being subjected to analysis by its own criteria. This set of values includes those of prediction, control, exploitation, and efficiency. It has been more recently argued that enlightenment naiveté in asserting the ability of science to produce value-free truths by value-free methods has failed (Seidman & Wagner, 1992). In other words, the foundational approach of the empirical analytic tradition as described by the logical positivists is an ideology.

Critical theorists argued that the assumption that fact and value can be separated implies that dealing only with facts is *better* than dealing with values because facts provide what is assumed to be an independent basis for distinguishing between theory and truth. This assumption also implies that dealing only with facts will produce outcomes for human beings that are *better* than outcomes produced by dealing with facts that have a value component.

Since foundationalism regards the world as a domain of neutral objects, foundational science is therefore prevented from examining itself as anything other than another neutral object, that is, without self-interest, or social origin, or values (Held, 1980). Foundational science thus submits every activity to causal analysis except its own (Allen, 1992).

In a crucial theoretical move, the critical theorists pointed out that the ideals of objectivity, efficiency, prediction, control, and value-freedom are themselves values. The notion that a true judgment (given that there is such a thing) is better than a false one is itself an evaluative statement (Held, 1980, p. 171). If science is indeed free of values, it follows that science is also free of ideological consequences. Thus, the assumption of value-freedom necessarily excludes inquiry into the possibility of the operation within science of systematic oppression through ideological means. Foundationalism thereby excludes consideration of the possibility that things might, under different circumstances, be different from how they are presently described by the scientific method (Seidman, 1992, p. 173). This is to say that positivist-based empirical analytic science excludes from rational inquiry the possibility of different meanings being attached to actions by the actors other than the meanings that are constructed by scientific activity.

In order to avoid the possibility of multiple interpretations, which would tend to destabilize the concepts under scrutiny, the meaning of concepts and methods in foundational science become reified. Methodological traditions are held apart from critique based on standards of ethical preferability, even when it has become apparent that they embody ideological deception and distortion (Seidman, 1992, p. 173) and oppression.

Foundationalism therefore reduces the concept of human agency to that of support or carrier of objective, measurable, value-free general social structures (Leonard, 1990). The critical theorists, however, pointed out that individuals can influence and are influenced by social structures. Seidman (1992), for example, observes the powerful effect of foundational science on people. Seidman argues that foundational science "promotes the intellectual obscurity and social irrelevance of theory, contributes to the decline of public morale and political discourse, and furthers the enfeeblement of an active citizenry" (p. 64). In other words, it is a disempowering ideology.

Certainly human behavior has indeed become regularized, predictable, controllable, and describable using sophisticated probability statistics and statistical modeling (Held, 1980). Under these conditions, social action does indeed appear to be governed by *natural* causal structures. But the use by the social sciences of the same approach found in the natural sciences on the *facts* of social life demonstrate an ironic truth. Instead of making the idea of human agency the subject of critical reflection, foundational methods tend to reify the structured consciousness of their constructed object. The observable is taken to be the only possibility, resulting in loss of context, history, possibility, and situatedness.

As an example of the unintended consequences of foundational science, consider the format of Sesame Street, the television program for preschool children in the United States. The structure of the program is based on research in psychology demonstrating that preschoolers learn best under certain circumstances, which include very short bursts of colorful, moving, anthropomorphic images repeated after a certain period of time. This research did not focus on the possibility that preschoolers *could learn* in other ways or *should learn* as they mature; rather, it focused only on how the sample *did learn* when measured by scientific observations based on foundational assumptions.

In structuring the program, this information was carefully followed without thought to the possibility of encouraging preschoolers to mature, that is, to have longer attention spans. Unfortunately, without challenge, preschoolers can remain at that stage of learning. Television programs for older children began to emulate the Sesame Street model in order to capture more viewers. MTV uses the same approach for teenagers, and the newspaper USA *Today* follows the same format for adults (Stewart & D'Angelo, 1988). The result is an entire generation of people who cannot follow any argument that lasts more than 40 seconds. The point is that the scientific description of learning among preschoolers not only *described* the normal, but also *produced* the normal without thought for the possible or the desirable.

Foundationalism has provided an extremely useful method to support technical and causal explanations for phenomena in the natural world. It is noted that what counts as the "natural world," however, is itself an ideological decision and should be recognized as such (Street, 1992). Technical reason is not problematic in itself. The problem is its use as a model for all valid knowledge and its categorical elimination of critique from any other perspective.

The foundational perspective survives in the natural sciences and the social sciences in various forms despite its widely acknowledged difficulties. The logical positivists were ultimately unable to determine the meaning of meaning, unable to define the essence of the concepts of verification, evidence, scientific explanation, and analysis, and unable to establish the *a priori* nature of mathematics and logic (Mish'alani, 1988, p. 4). The critique of foundationalism by the critical social theorists is shared by discourse analysis and other interpretive methodologies, although hybrid examples are forming (Denzin, 1997).

POSTMODERNISM

Another important influence on discourse analysis is the postmodern perspective. Postmodern theorists have criticized the critical social theorists with regard to their notion of transcendental concepts and the role of theory building. A modernist approach to science is one that assumes certain transcendental notions as a basis for theorizing. Foundational science is modernist in that the assumptions include certain transcendental notions such as the existence of "bare facts" and the "epistemological superiority of science as a mode of knowledge" (Seidman, 1992, p. 59).

Postmodernism, on the other hand, rejects totalizing narratives and universal reified concepts (even such concepts as domination or emancipation) in favor of situated accounts of a more local nature. It is an openly moral analysis that seeks to analyze specific contextual power relations by observing the processes of meaning-making that function within specific situations. Instead of analyzing the reified concepts illuminated by the process of the discourse, postmodernism analyzes the process itself.

Critical social theory has been called modernist by Leonard (1990) despite its critique of foundationalism because while it criticizes the transcendental notions of science, it makes use of other transcendental notions in the process. For example, critical social theory, while critical of the empirical analytic notion of a foundation of unassailable "true facts," assumes other notions to be universal, ahistorical, and transcendental. Critical social theory, for instance, assumes the notions of oppression, empowerment, and emancipation to be universal in the same sense as the notion of the existence of true facts.

The modernist project of critical social theory was designed to eliminate the ideological function of foundational science. However, in order to do so, critical social theory used what were assumed to be transcendentally valid principles, which could produce social reconstruction in emancipatory ways (Seidman & Wagner, 1992). The modernism of critical social theory therefore suffered from two incompatible self-imposed tasks: "being broad enough to encompass all human activity, and being specific enough to do this in a nontrivial way" (Nicholson, 1992, p. 83).

Leonard supports the claim that critical social theory is modernist with an important piece of evidence. Critical theorists believe that notions found in some nondominant discourses of modernity, such as Marxism, are sources of change strategies that can be reified and generalized to all human beings. The critical theorists criticized Marxist theory for universalizing emancipatory interest (and locating it in the proletariat) when they in fact committed a similar error themselves by insisting that their claims about more general domination, communication, and rationality had to be transcendental to be valid (Leonard, 1990). Anything less was too relativistic to be theoretically useful. Anything more would not be specific enough to be emancipatory. Critical theory can thus be viewed as another "interested" inquiry claiming universal truths from an unacknowledged situated position and therefore having the potential for unintended ideological consequences (Aronowitz, 1992).

On the positive side, modernism provided the important emphasis on historicity, possibility, and contextuality that was extended even further by the postmodernists such as discourse analysts. Postmodernists avoid postulating transcendental concepts (such as oppression or emancipation) as having an existence outside of specific human situations. Postmodernists do not assume theoretical constructs to have the logical status of natural laws.

Lowenberg (1993) points out that the postmodern influence has had observable effects across various approaches to inquiry such as phenomenology, hermeneutics, and symbolic interactionism. Among discourse analysts, Foucault, for example, rejects the possibility of a secure, objective, value-neutral foundation of empirical facts or transcendental universal social notions for the social sciences (Seidman & Wagner, 1992).

Instead of criticizing society from universal norms, postmodernists criticize universal norms from their context-specific social base (Alexander, 1992, p. 343). The postmodernist position "reconsider[s] the relationship between scientific knowledge, power and society as well as the relation between science, critique, and narrative" (Seidman & Wagner, 1992, p. 2).

Methodologically, "postmodernists prefer local stories to general ones, but do not necessarily reject methodologically sophisticated and analytically informed social analysis but rather invoke a suspicion regarding claims that social inquiry can be grounded in some way that gives it a privileged epistemological status" (Nicholson, 1992, p. 83). Postmodernists like Foucault are more likely to "do" history instead of theory building and to view moral and political concerns as central issues but not as transcendentally valid reified entities (Seidman & Wagner, 1992).

The postmodern tradition is described as narrative with moral intent (Seidman, 1992, p. 47). Postmodern discourse analysts refuse legitimation of research traditions in the social sciences that are based on discussions of "truth." Instead, the postmodern approach seeks to expand the numbers of people who may participate, since the intent is practical and openly moral. Local narratives claim to analyze social situations (AIDS, homelessness, and divorce, for example) in a particular social setting, while viewing the power relations inherent in the situation from a historical standpoint, in present circumstances, and for future possibilities (Seidman, 1992, p. 73).

FOUCAULT

Michel Foucault wrote in the tradition of the postmodernist extension of the critical social theorists' critique of the application of empirical analytic science to the human sciences. Foucault's work emphasizes the concept of power in specific human contexts. Any body of knowledge, any discipline in the human sciences that claims to produce definitions in its own area of expertise, is today faced with the observation that so-called "empirical" definitions change historically and discontinuously; that is, they do not reflect transcendental or universal subjects, meanings, structures, realities, or processes (Allen, 1986).

Accordingly, Wittgenstein had previously argued for treating all philosophical problems as manifestations of tensions between and within intra- and interdisciplinary discursive practices. According to Wittgenstein, philosophical issues should be understood as tensions between discursive practices, without demands for definitions or essences. Analysis of issues becomes a description of the discursive tensions in all of their concreteness and situatedness (Mish'alani, 1988, p. 4).

Foucault's work was not only influenced by this notion of the historical aspect of definitions and definition-producing discourse from Wittgenstein but also by the historical and power components of definitions from Nietzsche. For Nietzsche, an attempt at redefinition is seen as a strategy for access to hegemony or dominance of one discourse over others (Mish'alani, 1988). The act of defining or redefining something thus constitutes a move of power. The importance of power for Nietzsche was also reflected in Foucault's work.

Nietzsche argued that current usage of any concept consists of historical conglomerates, borrowings, dominations, plunderings, shifts, displacements, transpositions, and impositions (Mish'alani, 1988, p. 9). This swirling, "cotton candy" mix of threads in any discourse or body of knowledge can be patiently unwound in an analysis that Nietzsche called a genealogy. Following Nietzsche, Michel Foucault agreed that any attempt at analysis must be considered another interpretation, or another power domination, and also used the term *genealogy*.

For Foucault, it followed that discourse cannot be analyzed only in the present, because the power components and the historical components create such a tangled knot of shifting meanings, definitions, and interested parties over periods of time. Consequently, a discourse analysis must be seen at the same time from a genealogical perspective in Nietzsche's sense, a power analytic in Nietzsche's sense, and another historically situated, tension-analyzing discourse in Wittgenstein's sense.

Foucault claimed that power relations in modern western civilization can be represented as resulting from several key conceptual changes beginning around the 17th century (Dreyfus & Rabinow, 1983). The development of the physical sciences, the industrial revolution, and the rise of capitalist nation-states took place at the same time that philosophers were describing the humanist perspective. These well documented changes were accompanied, according to Foucault, by a gradual and generally unrecognized change in western practices of people management. Together, these reconceptualizations have reframed our modern assumptions concerning power, society, science, and the notion of human agency.

The emergence of the physical sciences freed our understanding of the physical world from traditional conceptualizations bound by religion and superstition. Before the scientific method, understanding of the physical world was based on magical thinking and/or faith handed down from traditional authorities such as legends and superstitions, official church teaching, or the divine authority of monarchs. There was a decidedly democratic goal associated with the developing empirical analytic method. Within the new method, truth claims became subject to replicable scrutiny following clearly defined rules that people could perform and observe themselves time after time. An important goal of the emerging physical sciences was control of the hardships of the natural environment. The impressive results in such areas as infection control and vaccination heralded the modern scientific epoch as we know it.

Concomitantly, the emergence of a philosophical perspective called *humanism* emphasized the liberty, equality, and fraternity of human beings (or at least a select group of people *defined* as human beings by those in positions of power—that is, White males). This philosophical orientation was contrasted with the traditional assumptions about people that held under religious monarchies. For example, the divine power of a king had formerly been understood to be absolute, and the interchangeable nature of any lesser person made it possible for the sovereign to exercise the divine right in any fashion that he or she so chose, usually involving external force. For example, a monarch might choose to make an example of someone caught poaching royal pheasants by public torture and death. The personal identity of the poacher had no meaning outside of the exercise of divine right. Within a humanist perspective, however, rudimentary notions of "natural rights" and "individual rights" began to emerge.

The best-documented change in western civilization during this time was the Industrial Revolution and the concurrent rise of capitalist economies. The mobilization of large groups of trained workers as a labor resource for capitalist economies became important for successful competition between nations. Continuity of this system requires stable groups of trained people that are reproduced in sufficient numbers. Capitalist economies are disrupted by large-scale migration, widespread famine or disease, and/or long-term warfare.

The gradual and steady replenishment of a docile and stable work force is therefore crucial to the emerging capitalist nation-state. Capitalism requires at least minimally trained people for industrial labor. People in the workforce are not as interchangeable as they were in feudal economies. This is to say that technical advice for the influence and control of individual human bodies and concern with the reproduction of workers became crucial to the success of capitalism.

In Foucault's view, these three conceptual changes are critical to understanding modern western civilization. Foucault adds another important change of perspective that has played a role in the determination of what modern life is like for those of us who live in it. Besides empirical analytic science, humanism, and capitalism, Foucault provides evidence for a shift in the conceptualization of power that is closely related to the three developments described previously. Based on Foucault's description of this shift in the conceptualization of power in modern western civilization, discourse analysis receives its impetus to describe power relations.

Several concepts organize Foucault's perspective and are important to understand when considering discourse analysis. These key concepts are power (also called bio-power in order to emphasize the important role of biology), resistance, the body, social science, social agents, and the medicalization and clinicalization of social control. These concepts exist at the societal level, according to Foucault, where they have come to function as cultural myths, ideologies, or unquestioned assumptions. Together, these concepts inform what Foucault calls a "strategy" that imparts direction to the micropractices of everyday life, as well as influencing larger social goals. Foucault calls this strategy bio-power or disciplinary power or power/knowledge.

Bio-power is concerned with the production of willing and able bodies that support the status quo of ongoing power relations, such as the economic system of capitalism. Foucault claims that this modern representation of power began as a mode of inquiry to answer specific questions about how to control people in certain specific situations. This approach was based on the success of control strategies used by foundational science on the natural world.

Before the 17th century, control of the minute details of human life had only taken place under extraordinary circumstances such as during outbreaks of plague, when, for example, people were confined to their houses in the evening and were physically counted by appointed citizens of the area. Around the 17th century, these successful measures of control were revisited and revised to meet new challenges in people control arising from the influence of capitalism and humanism. Applying the newly developed methods that were so successful in the physical sciences to problems concerning human beings generated by the rise of capitalism resulted in what is now called the social sciences. Foucault uses the terms *disciplinary technology, power/ knowledge*, and *human sciences* to refer to the social sciences in a manner that emphasizes the aspect of control of human beings adapted from the physical sciences.

Foucault claims that the conceptualization of power in modern society that has evolved from these developments in human rationality has become the assumed framework for understanding the notion of progress in western civilization. First developed and refined through specific practices applied to limited situations such as prisons and boarding schools, power and control practices became successful strategies applied in other situations such as law enforcement, hospitals, and schools. Discourse concerning how to build a better prison, how to enforce better military discipline, and how to build schools and hospitals was directed toward making them more efficient and therefore more successful. The same approach that emphasizes control was also applied to the education of children, the conduct of police, and the rules of order for large gatherings and meetings such as Robert's Rules of Order. These are all examples of approaches to the technology of social order that have this common ancestry or genealogy. The empirical analytic approach to the control of natural phenomena was successfully applied to the social world and linked with the progress of western civilization for the assumed definition of better outcomes for human beings.

These specific discourses of control were not discussed or debated as philosophies or theories per se. Instead, the discourses referred only to specific concrete situations, for example, "How should we build prisons so that we can see every inmate separately but prevent them from knowing when it is that they are being watched?" The work of the social sciences is carried out by members of the social disciplines educated within the framework of each discipline such as law enforcement, health care, sociology, psychology, and so on. The underlying and unaddressed order and control assumptions common to all of the social disciplines share the ancestry of the successful control of physical phenomena using empirical analytic science for the widely accepted goals of capitalism and the humanistic assumptions concerning the value and importance of individual human lives.

POWER

The following is an interpretation of Foucault's notion of the modern form of power in western civilization from all of the sources (both primary and secondary) that are listed in the reference section at the end of this chapter. The notion of power is the most important notion in Foucault's work because it forms the basis for the related concepts such as the analysis of discourse. The main exposition of the notion of power is found in Foucault's *The History of Sexuality, Volume One, Introduction* (1978), and the description provided here is mainly drawn from that account.

1. Power must be understood as a network of interacting forces that are goal-driven, relational, and self-organized. Power creates tensions between, within, and among individuals or groups. This is to say that power is not understood as a singular, unidirectional, reified phenomenon with identifiable instances of application. Power is not necessarily viewed as a strategy consciously used by some people over other people. Social life is viewed as a web of shifting power relations that changes through the processes of micropolitics and negotiation instead of brute physical force.
2. Power is a process that operates in continuous struggles and confrontations that change, strengthen, or reverse the polarity of the force relations between power and resistance. This means that power is described as a relational process that is embodied in context-specific situations and is partially identifiable through its ideological effects on the lives of people.
3. Power is the support that the force relations or tensions find in one another, forming a web or system of interacting influences. This is to say that wherever power is found, resistance to power is also found. For example, the domination of patriarchy is partially sustained by the definition of women as not-men. In other words, each is necessary to the other and each is defined in terms of the other. Each concept constitutes and is constituted by the other.
4. Power is the tension of the inherently contradictory relations between power and resistance. In other words, power can be partially described by the conflicting goals and objectives of power and resistance. This tension can only be described in specific terms relative to people in that situation and not in general terms that apply to other times and places.
5. Power is known from the strategies and practices in and through which the force relations take effect. One example of strategies and practices is the process of marginalization. Marginalization is the process by which nondominant discourses are not eliminated but tolerated as alternative speaking positions of resistance that provide the target and therefore the tension to sustain the dominant discourse. This process is necessary because power and resistance are defined in relation to

one another. The institutional manifestations of these strategies and practices of power may be found in bureaucracy, law, and various social hegemonic discourses such as science, medicine, and education. Power is not an ideology in Althusser's sense (1971), although ideology can be said to be one of the strategies seen within individual instances of domination in power relations.

For example, the ideology of capitalism is necessarily dependent on the existence of labor while at the same time marginalizing the voice of labor away from the process of decision making with respect to the production of capital. Marxist ideology provides a perspective that makes the social order understandable. It is also possible to use power relations as an alternative conceptual framework for understanding social order that includes the Marxist ideology as a specific instance of power relations. The grid or web of power relations described by Foucault constitutes an interpretation of social order arising from context-related practical concerns instead of theoretical necessity.

Power is not a group of institutions, a structure, or a set of mechanisms that ensures the subservience of citizens. Power is not a mode of subjugation functioning by rules instead of by violence. Instead, power functions through strategies and practices without conscious direction. Here Foucault means to distinguish his notion of power from the juridico-discursive notion of power prevalent in western philosophy and based on a notion of a democratically defined person with basic human rights in a sovereign-subject relation (Mish'alani, 1988).

Power is not a physical strength we are endowed with in some essentialist manner. Power does not mean a general system of domination by one group over another. In fact, Foucault emphasizes that situations of domination are embodied as much within the dominators as the oppressed. These individual instances of power usually called domination or oppression are effects, or terminal forms of power; they are points in the web or grid of power relations.

Power is not thought of as a negative restraint on truth or the rights of individuals or groups as it is conceptualized in the juridico-discursive view. Instead, power is *productive* of truth, rights, and the conceptualization of individuals. It is productive through the processes or discursive practices of the human sciences and other major discourses, including social sciences, medicine, penology, education, and psychiatry. Education within these discourses produces social agents who assume that scientific bodies of knowledge produce value-free truth, which advances western civilization by increasing the efficient management of human life and produces measurable outcomes, including happiness.

There is no central point from which all power emanates. Instead, power consists of a continually shifting web or grid of individual positions of tension between power and resistance. Because of the inequality of the tension, local and unstable states of power and resistance are constantly being created, dissolved, reversed, and reshuffled. Power is omnipresent not because it consolidates everything as arising from a unified source. It is omnipresent because it is continually produced in every relation from one moment to the next, in one situation to the next, between and among people in specific situations.

Power has a different complex strategical existence in the context of each particular manifestation. This strategical existence may be analyzed in its local effects without claims for universal application. Instead, the local strategy is described in terms of the local effects of domination on the individuals and groups involved. For example, the existence of power in an individual case of gender relations (a marriage, for instance) may be analyzed in terms of the limits that are placed on the actions of one or both of the participants.

Foucault sometimes refers to power as power/knowledge, because in discourse power and knowledge are joined together in relation to resistance. Discourse, therefore, may be both an instrument and an effect of both power and resistance. It transmits and produces power but also can undermine and expose it. Similarly, positions of silence can enact power but can also loosen the hold of power and provide obscure areas of tolerance for resistance. The most important level of analysis for power relations is at the level of micropractices—that is, the everyday activities of life which are the terminal points of the grid or web.

From this description of Foucault's approach to the subject of power, certain conclusions follow:

1. Power is not a reified finite entity that is acquired, seized, or shared. It is not something that someone can hold on to or allow to slip away. It is *embodied* or *performed* through the interplay of nonequal and changing relations of force in a specific context.
2. Power does not exist apart from economic relations, knowledge relations, or sexual relations; rather, it is inherent in them. Power is the immediate embodied effect of divisions and inequalities as they occur in context. Power has a direct productive role in these relations.
3. Power is not the institutionalized conflict between authorities and target groups. It does not proceed only in a top-down fashion. It functions in bureaucracy as well as in families, groups, institutions, discourses, and relationships. Larger scale lines of force are sometimes created out of the conglomeration of points in the power web, which can link points together and bring about redistributions. Major domination is the effect that is sustained when points in the grid are consolidated. Examples of these kinds of major dominations are described by Marxism and feminism with regard to class and gender, respectively.
4. Power relations are not intentional. There are directions to the lines of force, but the strategies are not necessarily planned to create oppression of specific people or groups. If power relations are understandable, it is not because they are an example of something that "explains" them but because they have common goals and objectives. These goals and objectives are only rarely identifiable as

related to power. More often than not, the goals and objectives are specified with respect to micropractices and have power effects as unintended consequences. The goals and objectives of an occupational therapist, for example, are not often thought of as related to power but instead are thought to function for the social and personal benefit of individual clients. Power effects of the relationship between the occupational therapist and the client can also be identified, however, and may be very instructive to the participants. The methods and the outcomes sought by the occupational therapist have been standardized by the discourse of occupational therapy but are not intentionally designed to produce power for the therapist.

Therefore, it cannot be said that power relations necessarily result from the choice or decision of an individual person or group of people. In fact, Foucault argues that modern power is not some sort of conspiracy set up with respect to specific goals of control. He calls his conceptualization of power a strategy without a strategist; though it provides direction for the ordering of power/ knowledge, no organized body of knowledge can be said to have originated the strategy.

The logic, order, or strategy of power is characterized by practices that often seem quite explicit at a restricted level, such as the design of classrooms with the teacher in front and the students facing forward. The logic of the system can be analyzed, and the aims can be completely understandable, and yet no one can be said to have specifically designed the logic to be oppressive. The overall strategy was constructed historically but not intentionally.

5. Wherever there is power, there is resistance that is implicit to the situation.

RESISTANCE

Resistance plays the role of adversary, target and/or support for power. Power and resistance both constitute and are constituted by each other. They are each defined by reference to one another. Thus, power and resistance are found together in all points of the web of power relations. The diversity of resistances is each a special case in relation to domination in that situation.

Resistance, like power, can coalesce to form large rebellions or radical ruptures such as the Civil Rights Movement of the 1960s in the United States. Resistance can also remain isolated in specific circumstances such as one workplace. Resistance works against power and can shift the tensions and create new alliances and fractures. Resistance can also be co-opted, or absorbed, by power in any force relation. Co-optation of resistance results in the increase of power and the reduction and/or fracturing of the resistance. An example of co-optation can be found in the absorption of doctors of osteopathy into the medical model.

Foucault believed it to be instructive to look at marginalized practices and discourses that are minimally exploited and controlled. He suggested looking for practices that have not been co-opted, or localized points of resistance, in order to shed light on the forms of oppression, potential subject positions, and empowering strategies that may exist in that context. Foucault did not claim that oppressed resistance strategies or speaking positions were in any way "better" than the oppressive dominant positions with which they coexist. Examining a marginalized practice such as herbal remedies, for example, is inherently problematic because studying them causes the ideology of science to be applied to them. Description begins the process of co-optation and control through normalization.

BIO-POWER

Foucault's work describes the form of power in our modern discursive epoch as *bio-power* or *power/knowledge*. Foucault's notion of bio-power is an interpretation of modernity arising from practical, not theoretical, concerns. He acknowledged that competing interpretations are possible and even likely. He specifically refers to bio-power as the social control of human affairs through the "normalizing strategies" of western social science. According to Foucault, the technical and instrumental rationality of foundational empirical analytic science that was used in such an exploitive and successful manner against the hardships of nature has become the model for all knowledge and truth in modern western civilization. The extension of empirical control to humans through the social sciences by disciplined social agents is a wide-ranging strategy-without-a-strategist that now affects everyone in western European-based cultures. Furthermore, the modern concept of power functions as an ideology that is an invisible cultural assumption common to all descriptions of progress. The concepts' invisibility is addressed by the notion of the repressive hypothesis.

THE REPRESSIVE HYPOTHESIS

The repressive hypothesis is a concept in Foucault's work that is an unintended consequence of bio-power. Foucault's notion of the repressive hypothesis was influenced by "Nietzsche's genealogy of the way power uses the illusion of meaning to further itself" (Dreyfus & Rabinow, 1983, p. xxvii). Nietzsche's work demonstrated how the illusion of meaning supports control strategies without the necessity of an appeal to the notion of an organized conspiracy. Foucault called this illusion of meaning, this ideology, the *repressive hypothesis*.

According to Foucault, the repressive hypothesis is the widely held assumption that the normalizing control of social science aids the progress of civilization because it produces value-free, objective truth. Foucault called this notion the repressive hypothesis because it engenders a noncritical attitude among people with respect to the authority of scientific truth. This cultural myth results in a kind of faith in science. For example, people assume that freely accessible scientific knowledge keeps authorities from having unchecked power over ordinary people (Dreyfus & Rabinow, 1983).

The repressive hypothesis can be said to function as one of the ideological consequences of the functioning of bio-power. It is ultimately in the interests of an ever-expanding role of control to increasing instances of daily life that the repressive hypothesis be widely assumed. In this way, the repressive hypothesis resembles the false consciousness of Marxist theory. However, in Foucault's case, there is no "true" consciousness because alternate representations can also be argued.

Under bio-power and the repressive hypothesis, technical, instrumental, means-end reasoning has been raised to the level of a social principle (Aronowitz, 1992, p. 302). Radical ideas that advocate resistance to the scientific management of everyday life are unfettered but unheard, because they seem so illogical, irrational, nonsensical, disorderly, uncivilized, and unscientific. Persuasion is not a method, but a content (p. 309). Persuasion is openly a discourse concerning compliance with the normalized truth of social science as the definition of *progress* in western civilization. Because of the repressive hypothesis, rejecting science is believed to be rejecting rationality. Human beings feel more and more coerced and controlled but have no target to which to direct concerns because of the constraints of scientifically determined normal behavior. Who can object to truth? Doesn't truth set you free? Doesn't more research, more truth, mean a better life for everyone?

CONFESSION

Another related aspect of social science for Foucault is the creation of self-revealing subjects by confession of personal truth to social agents viewed as authorities. The act of confession and the repressive hypothesis both support the functioning of the modern conceptualization of power. According to Foucault, the confession of personal truth serves a social function that has become an obsession in our modern existence (Dreyfus & Rabinow, 1983). Social agents, those representatives of science-based disciplines, are educated in their roles as evaluators of revealed truth.

Confession has served as a model for the provision of health care. Individuals who reveal truths about themselves to social authorities believe the process to be therapeutic because it allows authorities to compare them to scientifically determined normal ranges and to take action. For example, patients allow their cholesterol levels to be measured so that medical science can intervene and adjust the levels to the normal range. We all believe this practice to be beneficial.

Confession is thus not a practice limited to religion or psychiatry but a more general practice that can be identified in discourses such as found in education, sociology, nursing, medicine, and popular culture in the form of call-in shows and self-help books. In nursing, confession occurs during the assessment phase of the nursing process. Clients confess to the nurse as a social agent and expect that the nurse will compare their truths to the normalized truth of nursing science and help them "get better" or "prevent illness."

THE BODY

Foucault emphasized the human body as the physical "space" for the operation of the social micropractices associated with the concepts of bio-power, resistance, confession, and the repressive hypothesis. "In the discursive history of strategies for making ourselves visible, knowable, and speakable, we have made great use of the metaphor of the body as a source of health and order, illness and disorder" (O'Neill, 1986, p. 352). In dominant patriarchal discourses such as medicine, the target is often the female body (McNay, 1992; Ussher, 2000).

Bodies can be considered terminal points in the web or grid of power relations between power/knowledge and resistance (Doering, 1992) and the site of social action, power, and resistance.

Much of the knowledge about human bodies that is represented as universal, value-free, ahistorical truth is more accurately described as a power/knowledge system specific to bodies, relative to historical time, inflected with the values and morals of the time and influenced by existent power structures. (Allman, 1991, p. 3)

The process of increasing control of individual bodies includes the use of discourses that create individual bodies as objects. Parents are influenced by "neutral, scientific" observations of their children such as descriptions of normal ranges and the ordering of individuals along the graded scale. Advice is sought concerning how to raise a "normal, well-adjusted" child. The emphasis on the individual as an object turns attention away from the strategy used to produce the light that shines to illuminate this object. Attention is thus directed to the illuminated object and not to the process of influence, the disciplinary power. In the process of constructing the knowledge that creates people's bodies as objects, people are convinced that speaking about themselves is important, even critical, to their own health and happiness and therefore to the overall good of society.

MEDICALIZATION AND CLINICALIZATION OF SOCIAL CONTROL

Two processes, the medicalization and the clinicalization of social control (O'Neill, 1986, p. 353), serve to illustrate the power relations among bio-power, the repressive hypothesis, confession, medicine, nursing, and bodies.

These connections facilitate understanding the role of discourse in nursing as participating in the expansion of the bio-power strategy of scientific control through normalization.

The medicalization of social control is visible when "system" problems of order and deviance in a culture begin to be addressed in terms of the medical model of disease and thereby bypass other discourses such as those of aesthetics and ethics. Human problems are not seen as social issues for discussion and critique but "problems" to be solved in terms of a diagnosis and treatment model.

In the process of medicalization, institutions are reified as systems and not as communities of people. In addition, interactive human relations become "outcomes," and "diagnoses" replace human situations in a moral, social context. Science is then applied for its technical control of these technical problems that have been stripped of contextual, ethical, and human dimensions. Social relations begin to be described in terms formerly used for object relations.

In this manner, the process of medicalization uses "body words" in a scientific way that assumes the terms are value-free, eliminates critique, promotes control, and assumes the desirability of its own results. Examples of body words include *maladaptation, minimal brain dysfunction, hyperactivity,* and *genetic.* For example, violence has recently been called a "public health epidemic." Such a definition completely denies the complex social context in favor of a medical "disease" approach. Sociobiology provides a similar example of the use of body words for social problems (see Rushton & Bogaert, 1989, with commentary by Leslie, 1990). The advantage, of course, in describing social problems in terms of disease is that while many sources of funds are currently available to treat diseases, there is very little money to address moral problems.

The discursive strategy of clinicalization functions in conjunction with medicalization. If the problems of social order and deviance are phrased in terms of medical diagnoses, then the "treatment" of such problems must occur on bodies in a physically medical space—that is, a clinical setting ordered by the authority of social agents that include nurses and doctors.

Clinical thinking in medicine thus occurs in the context of medicine's position as a discourse not based on a concept of personal identity but on the existence of the human body as a space to be acted upon (Scott, 1987). Indeed, Foucault argues that medicine arose as a linguistic reorganization of the concept of disease within the space of the body, utilizing the "ordering theoretical gaze" of the authority, the physician. This theoretical reorganization constitutes what Foucault calls one of the historical conditions of possibility for the discourse of medicine (Foucault, 1975).

For example, the changing health care system in the United States has the potential to change the traditional focus of medical discourse applied to the space of the human body. Fee for service medical care is being replaced with continuous payments to insurance companies. In the former system, profit occurs when people are treated for illnesses; in the latter system, profit occurs when people stay healthy, keep making their insurance payments, and do not need health care. In this latter system, health care systems keep more of the money they make if they keep people healthy. When money is made by keeping people healthy, the processes of medicalization and clinicalization will turn to addressing health as the clinical condition to be treated so that more money can be made. Prevention becomes the control strategy, and illnesses will be treated as system failures.

The closely related processes of medicalization and clinicalization serve to protect and enlarge the current social domination by medical science. Time, space, and discourse are not transcendental concepts; instead, they inhabit individual bodies and populations directly, informing our perceptions, perceived limits, options, and approaches (Scott, 1987). The conceptual ordering of the physical space of the body can be created or dissolved over time for different purposes, such as the creation of new discourses and their related discursive practices.

SOCIAL SCIENCE AND THE ROLE OF SOCIAL AGENTS

The social sciences constitute people as meaningful subjects and docile objects at the same time. This means that the notion of a person is constructed to be someone who speaks her or his experience and complies with social agents in order to obtain the proper "normal" outcomes. The control of biopower is evidenced by the process of "normalizing" individuals with respect to standards set through social science based on the foundational assumptions inherent in the empirical analytic method. Confession creates speaking individuals who can be influenced by social agents through comparison to the normalized scientific truth. This normalized truth is produced and applied by the social agents to people.

For example, the emphasis on *assessment* in many disciplines, including nursing, makes use of speaking subjects in order to compare what the person being assessed says to the normal version described in the body of scientific knowledge ordered by the discipline. Assessment is performed with the purpose of comparison to normal, and intervention is initiated to produce movement in the direction of standards of "normal." These standards are often given the even more scientific word *outcomes*, which takes the concept further away from any notion of variation.

The truth produced by social science is widely believed to be in the best interests of advancing civilization in the direction of individual freedom due to increasingly informed choice. This belief is an aspect of the repressive hypothesis. However, Foucault argues that the production of truth in this manner serves instead to decrease or limit options for informed choice by individuals. The options are limited because scientific narratives describe "the way things are" or the "natural categories" that do not change, despite the acknowledged imperfections in any current scientific description. Theoretically, one is able to "choose" from many options. Unfortunately, many options now have a social stigma of scientific unacceptability.

For example, the descriptions of "naturally male" behavior in conversation depicted in popular books (using the analogy of males and females as originating from different planets) serves to effectively reduce any tendency a woman may have had to identify with or display any of the "male" traits, and vice versa. People have the choice, but who would choose something that is associated with the other gender? Diversity is reduced by "objective" descriptions produced by scientific methods and generalized to entire populations from a limited sample. When faced with the statement that "most women do X," few males would consciously choose to do X.

Social agents have become responsible for dissemination of the results of truth-producing discourses in a manner that ensures understanding and compliance. Social agents include bureaucrats, police, teachers, nurses, doctors, lawyers, and other members of disciplines that employ a body of knowledge, or a discourse. Since the results are considered to be "true" because they were generated by the scientific methodology, then the news must be spread far and wide so that people have choices in a democratic society and are not prevented from knowing "the truth." The daily newscast may report preliminary results from a study published that very day in the *New England Journal of Medicine*, whether it is a pilot study or a full-blown clinical trial.

Science is expensive and time consuming and can only be supported by a dominant ideology. The asking of questions, the formulation of methods, the recruitment of subjects, the analysis of data, and the statement of conclusions all assume the value-free nature of scientific activity. The truth that is revealed cannot be absolute in any sense, because there is no position outside of our own situated perspective from which to evaluate a truth that is said to be "human nature."

According to Foucault, an important result of the proliferation of such technical social knowledge is the expansion of bureaucracy to administer more detailed programs, to gather more information, and to monitor progress and compliance. This necessitates the addition of more social agents and the extension of institutions in which to educate them. Large-scale funding and dissemination of scientific research on human beings and their environment is used to describe increasingly finer details of physical, psychological, and social "facts." The role of social agent, or expert, is widely assumed to be necessary to maintain social order and is considered to be a desirable position with elevated status, monetary reward, and power. The role of social agent is considered by those who are not members to be a sellout to "the establishment." Supervisors, bureaucrats, doctors, lawyers, and politicians are all considered by others to be "them" instead of "us," even though their power, money, and influence are envied and desired and their positions are considered necessary. Everyone, however, is a "them" to some of "us."

The social sciences are considered important because of the necessity of continued advances in individuals and groups as objects of study and as speaking subjects. More information (in increasingly finer detail) is critical for tighter description and therefore better social management and better outcomes for everyone. Administrative people are necessary to manage individuals and populations through surveillance by the methods of social science.

Over time, the amount of surveillance needed to produce control decreases as people internalize more of the results of the truth about human beings and "know" more about themselves as a result of speaking as subjects. This enables the extant machinery of science and bureaucracy to shift to some related topic that requires more research. It does not seem to enable the existing apparatus to become any smaller.

The mechanism of surveillance itself becomes less crucial in late welfare capitalism. Self-control is achieved by incomplete surveillance, a principle of operant conditioning. For example, consider traffic control. Your behavior in traffic is not continually monitored, but the threat of being "caught" keeps the driver from committing offenses most of the time.

Social science produces "true" descriptions of the behavior of groups and individuals. Normal ranges and outliers can then be identified. Categories can be amalgamated or split and redefined as necessary according to evolving scientific truth. Knowing more about people makes it easier to influence people, to manage order, and to create economic progress. People internalize the importance of science and readily volunteer for studies to find out more about themselves by becoming speaking subjects. Normal values then become the standard, and careful measurements on individuals can determine their position in the normal range. For example, schools, military, police, and the medical profession all make use of observation (surveillance) in this sense.

An excellent example of this kind of influence (graciously provided by K. Allman) is the "truth" of the Metropolitan Life Insurance height and weight tables. This information is carefully researched, compiled, published, and sent free to physicians' offices to be prominently displayed. Also used in the calculation of life insurance rates, this information finds its way into magazines and other public media, where people can compare their own height and weight to that of the table. Diet counseling can be based on such data. Adequacy of nutrition for marginalized groups can be assessed using such data. Egos are strained or stroked by comparison to such normalized truth. Later, this "truth" can be redefined according to the up-to-the-minute figures that might change any of the numbers on the chart. To your surprise, you find that you were in the normal range last year, but according to the new figures, you weigh too much. Has truth changed?

The observations and descriptions of the human sciences are conducted with full public knowledge and even celebration of important findings. No one objects to the description of normal, to the creation of categories, or to the assignment of persons to categories. On the contrary, as soon as descriptive results become public, people tend to compare themselves to the information and find a place for themselves in the schema. For example, consider the visual learner versus the auditory learner versus the hands-on learner. Everyone tries to decide where they fit. People then base decisions on what kind of learner they are without considering what kind of learner they could be or should be. The systematic manipulation of categories of people seems entirely rational, positive, and scientific. Simple description becomes intervention because it carries the weight of scientific truth and because the importance of social order and progress have been internalized with the help of the repressive hypothesis. We measure our subjective worth as humans depending on our place in a published schematic.

It seems quite unthinkable to object to the advancement of scientific truth. The point here is that it is taken for granted that this perspective will increase the quality of life for human beings, or at least for those defined as human beings. As an example of this kind of thinking, Foucault points to a contradiction dating from the 19th century. At that time, anthropology claimed that the incest taboo was universal among human beings. At the same time, however, there were extensive government programs in place to eradicate the practice in lower class and rural locations. In other words, now that we have this normalized truth, we had better get out there and make sure everyone conforms to it. This process will inevitably use a lot of time, money, and personnel.

As another example (provided by D. Allen), consider why such massive efforts are presently being proposed and mobilized to prop up the institution of the family if "the family" is such a natural thing to begin with? If so many people are not staying in traditional family groupings, why is it necessary to try and reconstruct a normalized truth? Is it really that "natural" after all?

The philosophical and methodological foundations of discourse analysis are applicable to many situations in nursing. As a method of inquiry, discourse analysis has the potential to inform nursing research and nursing practice. The method of producing a discourse analysis has been briefly described elsewhere (Powers, 1996). Awareness and understanding of power and oppression in nursing discourses could benefit from the use of this method.

REFERENCES

Alexander, J. (1992). General theory in the postpositivist mode: The 'epistemological dilemma' and the search for present reason. In S. Seidman & D. Wagner (Eds.), *Postmodernism and social theory*. Cambridge, MA: Blackwell.

Allen, D. (1985). Nursing research and social control: Alternative models of science that emphasize understanding and emancipation. *Image, 17*, 58–64.

Allen, D. (1986). Using philosophical and historical methodologies to understand the concept of health. In P. Chinn (Ed.), *Nursing research methodology* (pp. 157–168). Rockville, MD: Aspen.

Allen, D.G. (1992). Feminism, relativism, and the philosophy of science: An overview. In J.L. Thompson, D.G. Allen, & L. Rodrigues-Fisher (Eds.), *Critique, resistance, and action: Working papers in the politics of nursing*. New York: NLN.

Allman, K.M. (1991). Theories of the body: Situated knowledges and critical narratives. In D. Allen, K.M. Allman & P. Powers, *Taken for Grantedness in Nursing*. Melbourne, Australia: Deakin University Press.

Allman, K.M. (1992). Race, racism, and health: Examining the 'natural' facts. In J. L. Thompson, D. G. Allen, & L. Rodrigues-Fisher (Eds.), *Critique, resistance, and action: Working papers in the politics of nursing*. New York: NLN.

Althusser, L. (1971). Ideology and ideological state apparatuses. In *Lenin and Philosophy*. New York: Modern Reader.

Aronowitz, S. (1992). The tensions of critical theory: Is negative dialectics all there is? In S. Seidman & D. Wagner (Eds.), *Postmodernism and social theory*. Cambridge, MA: Blackwell.

Cheek, J. (1997). Negotiating delicately: Conversations about health. *Health and Social Care in the Community*, 5(1), 23–27.

Cheek, J., & Rudge, T. (1994). Inquiry into nursing as textually mediated discourse. In P. Chinn (Ed.), *Advances in methods of inquiry for nursing* (pp. 59–67). Gaithersburg, MD: Aspen.

DeMarco, R., Campbell, J., & Wuest, J. (1993). Feminist critique: Searching for meaning in research. *Advances in Nursing Science*, 16(2), 16–38.

Denzin, N.K. (1997). *Interpretive ethnography: Ethnographic practices of the 21st* century. Thousand Oaks, CA: Sage.

Doering, L. (1992). Power and knowledge in nursing: A feminist poststructuralist view. *Advances in Nursing Science*, 14(4), 24–33.

Dreyfus, H. (1987). Foucault's critique of psychiatric medicine. *Journal of Medicine and Philosophy*, 12(4), 311–333.

Dreyfus, H., & Rabinow, P. (1983). *Michel Foucault, beyond structuralism and hermeneutics*. Chicago: University of Chicago Press.

Dzurec, L. (1989). The necessity for and evolution of multiple paradigms for nursing research: A poststructuralist perspective. *Advances in Nursing Science*, 11(4), 69–77.

Foucault, M. (1975). *The birth of the clinic*, (A. M. Sheridan-Smith, Trans.). New York: Vintage/Random House.

Foucault, M. (1978, 1985, 1986). *The History of Sexuality* (Vols. 1, 2, and 3, Robert Hurley, Trans.). New York: Random House.

Gavey, N. (1997). Feminist poststructuralism and discourse analysis. In M. Gergen & S.N. Davis (Eds.), *Toward a new psychology of gender* (pp. 49–63). New York: Routledge.

Gray, P. (1999, October). *Feminist methodology: Preconference workbook*. Tenth Annual Critical and Feminist Inquiry in Nursing Conference, Williamsburg, Virginia.

Habermas, J. (1971). *Knowledge and human interests*. Boston: Beacon Press.

Hedin, B. A. (1986). A case study of oppressed group behavior in nurses. *Image*, 18(2), 53–57.

Held, D. (1980). *Introduction to critical theory*. Berkeley: University of California Press.

Hinshaw, A.S., Feetham, S.L. & Shaver, J.L.F. (Eds.). (1999) *Handbook of clinical nursing research*. Thousand Oaks, CA: Sage.

Kusch, M. (1991). *Foucault's strata and fields: An investigation into archaeological and genealogical science studies*. Dordrecht, The Netherlands: Kluwer Academic Publishers.

Leonard, S. T. (1990). *Critical theory in political practice.* Princeton: Princeton University Press.

Leslie, C. (1990). Scientific racism: Reflections on peer review, science and ideology. *Social Science and Medicine,* 31(3), 891–912.

Lowenberg, J.S. (1993). Interpretive research methodolgy: Broadening the dialogue. *Advances in Nursing Science,* 16(2), 57–69.

Lupton, D. (1992). Discourse analysis: A new methodology for understanding the ideologies of health and illness. *Australian Journal of Public Health* 16, 145-150.

McNay, L. (1992). *Foucault and Feminism.* Boston: Northeastern University Press.

Mish'alani, J. K. (1988). *Michel Foucault and philosophy: An overview.* Unpublished paper. University of Washington at Seattle.

Nicholson, L. (1992). On the postmodern barricades: Feminism, politics, and theory. In S. Seidman & D. Wagner (Eds.), *Postmodernism and social theory.* Cambridge, MA: Blackwell.

O'Neill, J. (1986). The medicalization of social control. *Canadian Review of Sociology and Anthropology,* 23(3), 350–364.

Passmore, J. (1967). Logical positivism. In Paul Edwards (Ed.), *The encyclopedia of philosophy, Volume Five* (pp. 52–57). New York, Macmillan.

Powers, P. (1996). Discourse analysis as a methodology for nursing inquiry. *Nursing Inquiry,* 3, 207–217.

Rushton, J. P., & Bogaert, A. F. (1989). Population differences in susceptibility to AIDS: An evolutionary analysis. *Social Science and Medicine,* 28(12), 1211–1220.

Scott, C. (1987). The power of medicine, the power of ethics. *Journal of Medicine and Philosophy,* 12(4), 334–350.

Seidman, S. (1992). Postmodern social theory as narrative with a moral intent. In S. Seidman & D. Wagner (Eds.), *Postmodernism and social theory.* Cambridge, MA: Blackwell.

Seidman, S., & Wagner, D. (Eds.). (1992). *Postmodernism and social theory.* Cambridge, MA: Blackwell.

Stepan, N. L. (1993). Race and gender: The role of analogy in science. In S. Harding (Ed.), *The racial economy of science: Towards a democratic future* (pp. 359–376). Bloomington; IN: Indiana University Press.

Stewart, J., & D'Angelo, G. (1988). *Together: communicating interpersonally* (3rd ed.). New York: Random House.

Street, A. F. (1992). *Inside nursing, a critical ethnography of clinical nursing practice.* Albany, NY: State U. of NY Press.

Thompson, J. L. (1985). Practical discourse in nursing: Going beyond empiricism and historicism. *Advances in Nursing Science,* 7 (4), 59–71.

Thompson, J. L. (1987). Critical scholarship: The critique of domination in nursing. *Advances in Nursing Science,* 10(1), 27–38.

Thompson, J. L. (1992). Identity politics, essentialism, and constructions of 'home' in nursing. In J. L. Thompson, D. G. Allen, & L. Rodrigues-Fisher (Eds.), *Critique, resistance, and action: Working papers in the politics of nursing.* New York: NLN.

Ussher, J. (2000). Women's madness: A material-discursive-intrapsychic approach. In W. Fee (Ed.), *Pathology and the postmodern* (pp. 207–230). London: Sage.

CHAPTER 2

THE FEMINIST CONTRIBUTION TO DISCOURSE ANALYSIS

INTRODUCTION

Discourse analysis as described and performed by Foucault participates in the critique of foundationalism and emphasizes the power component in situated discourses. Although Foucault's work rarely mentioned power relations between men and women, work has been done to apply the Foucaultian perspective to gender relations. In the process, feminist theorists have clarified and extended Foucault's work. "What Foucault's work offers feminists, however, is a contextualization of experience and an analysis of its constitution and ideological power" (Weedon, 1987, p. 125). This chapter will describe feminist positions with regard to power and how these positions have influenced discourse analysis.

THE CRITIQUE OF EMPIRICAL ANALYTIC SCIENCE

The scientific method described in the 16th century was believed to be what the church was not, that is, value neutral and free of politics and social influences (Riger, 1992). The assumptions of empirical analytic science have been disputed by critical social theory and postmodernist critiques as described in chapter 1.

Most philosophers of science had widely assumed that a general theory concerning the nature of knowledge was possible. More recently, however, feminists have agreed with critical theorists and postmodernists, arguing that there are good reasons to question this assumption (Alcoff & Potter, 1993). Knowledge is not value neutral at all; instead, it serves as ideology, as an organizing social myth. In this view, knowledge is deeply political, functioning to legitimize and reinforce the current power arrangements (Harding, 1986).

Philosophical supporters of empirical analytic science do not, however, acknowledge its social origin, claiming that because of its objectivity, it can and should submit everything to analysis. Some feminists have argued that scientific knowledge is masculine and therefore inherently designed to address morally driven class- and power-based projects (Harding, 1986). This view holds that if the word *ideology* were substituted for *science*, and if *power* were substituted for *truth*, then the process of knowledge development would have more insight into its own functioning.

Consider the empirical analytic literature concerning biological femaleness. The initial underlying motivation for research into the biology of women was to discover *why* it was "natural" for women to be and function in society the way that they do (Hubbard, 1990). One unintended consequence of this perspective, for example, is that the completely normal processes of menstruation and menopause have become defined as medical diseases that should be treated by medical technologies. Medically, menstruation is viewed as the failure of a baby, and menopause is the failure of femininity (Martin, 1997). The "joke" goes as follows: Never trust anything that can bleed for five days and still live. "Not bleeding" is assumed to be the biological normal, and women are measured against that normal. Since men do not bleed for five days every month (nor do girls, menopausal women, pregnant women, and many normal women) bleeding must be something abnormal and should not be trusted by any normal person. Woman is the theoretical other, alternatively considered better or worse but never analogous (Tavris, 1992).

Biological language always has been metaphorical. Martin (1991), for example, has analyzed the words used to describe biological processes. Women *shed* eggs, while men *produce* sperm. Words used for the behavior of sperm cells are all masculine. They are *strong*, they *lurch*, they *penetrate*, and they *journey in quest of the ovum*; egg cells, on the other hand, *drift* along the fallopian tubes. Recent research has shown that the egg has a much more aggressive role, but the descriptive terms remain feminine and passive (Martin, 1991).

Martin (1997) also has analyzed the controversial theory concerning the role of menstruation in removing viral and bacterial pathogens brought into the uterus by sperm cells. She concludes that the vehemence of the debate can be explained not by the hypothesis of a more active role of the uterus in the immune system but by the implication that sperm cells can carry harmful particles.

Feminism has pointed out that biological metaphors of difference for any groups that are not White and/or male have become diagnostic and function as essential characteristics of a group of people. Consider that there is no good scientific evidence that African Americans are more "at risk" of hypertension than European Americans *because of their skin color* (Kaufman & Cooper, 1995). And yet most nursing textbooks repeat this unsupported assertion. Metaphors of similarity are rare (Stepan, 1993), because research that supports a hypothesis of "no difference" is not publishable. Research that supports any differences between imaginary categories of people creates and/or perpetuates the inferiority of one of them.

One of the unintended consequences of using metaphors of difference is that it marginalizes groups of people (Hall, Stevens, & Meleis, 1994). Marginalization is defined as "the process through which persons are peripheralized on the basis of their identities, associations, experiences, and environments" (Hall et al., 1994, p. 25). Groups such as inner city homeless people, Native Americans, and unmarried mothers are marginalized by dominant discourses found in professional disciplines and repeated in the media, political arenas, popular writing, and so on. Nursing research that focuses on marginalized groups has only recently appeared (see Hall, 1994). Nursing research on single parent families, for instance, has categorized them as *broken, deviant, incomplete, pathological*, and *less functional* (Ford-Gilboe & Campbell, 1996).

Worth (1997) has pointed out the serious consequences of marginalizing discourse in her analysis of a 1993 case against an African man in New Zealand who was HIV-positive. The man was charged with willful infection of sexual partners. The discourse within the courtroom and in the media concerned the man as Black, compared to his sexual partners who were White. The public discourse then used his marginal status as the basis for calls for exclusionary laws against Black people instead of focusing on the dangers of unprotected sex.

Similarly, power/knowledge has essentialized the concept of aggression to the definition of men and not to the essential definition of women. Female warriors, for example, in certain Native American tribes were completely ignored in early descriptions of American Indians (Blackwood, 1993). Parallel to the biological language, U.S. culture has eroticized both dominance and submission. The feminization of romantic love, for example, was a gradual social discursive process that took place in Europe beginning in the Middle Ages (Cancian, 1993).

Nowhere is the discursively constructed "normal" aggressive and violent essence of men more clear and more accepted as fact than in the case of rape. Aggression is so central to the definition of man that defining rape is actually viewed as a legal problem. MacKinnon (1987) points out that the crime of rape centers around the male concept of penetration. The use of this concept explains why there are problems defining marital rape (because a wife is a man's "property" that he regularly penetrates) and rape of women who are not virgins (because clearly they have "nothing" to lose). Loss of dignity does not apply in the male (legal) definition of rape.

Law is described by MacKinnon as masculine in the same manner as empirical analytic science in that both western social institutions assume that they reflect 'what is.' The law defines rape by the male standard of *behavior* instead of by the victim's threshold of *consent* or point of violation. Consent is not a meaningful concept in the legal definition of rape. "From whose standpoint, and in whose interest, is a law that allows one person's conditioned unconsciousness to contraindicate another's experienced violation?. . . rewarding men with acquittals for not comprehending women's point of view on sexual encounters" (MacKinnon, 1987, p. 146).

The violent essence of men is a legal "fact," an excuse, and an explanation. Consequently, from the perpetrator's point of view, the only risk in rape is "getting caught" (Scully & Marolla, 1993). On the other hand, perpetrators report the rewards of rape to be significant. One perpetrator told the female of this pair of researchers, "Rape is a man's right. If a woman doesn't want to give it, the man should take it. Women have no right to say no." (Scully & Marolla, 1993, p. 410).

The feminist critique of essentializing empirical analytic science is well documented. What to do with the critique is not. Harding (1986) argues that we need not abandon rational discourse as a result of the feminist critiques of science. Instead, we need to strengthen rationality and apply it to the very basis of science, problematizing the assumptions on which it stands. Discourse analysis is a strategy that can be extremely useful in this task. Unfortunately, women have been denied the opportunity to generate knowledge unless they claim objectivity and follow the rules of empirical analytic science, thus simply producing more male oriented knowledge. Hubbard (1990, p. 29) therefore argues that feminists must instead draw attention to the technologies that dominant groups use to deny marginalized groups the power to make facts in the ways that they do.

From this perspective, feminist research works to de-center the perspective of the essentialized White Anglo-Saxon male (Denzin, 1997). Decentralizing dominant discourses is not easy, however, because discourses tend to take on a life of their own. For example, physical anthropology abandoned the project of classifying different races among the human species long ago, yet biomedical science and epidemiology still use the concept of race in research (Kaufman & Cooper, 1995).

Harding (1986) has described different feminist epistemologies used to critique the assumptions of foundational science. She describes three types of feminist epistemologies: feminist empiricist philosophy, feminist standpoint theory, and feminist postmodernist philosophy. Feminist empiricist philosophy (also called liberal feminism) purports to construct "equal" knowledge from the singular perspective of women's lives using the same methods as traditional empirical analytic science. Liberal feminist empiricism assumes that truly objective science will overcome the bias toward men and will result in gender-fair knowledge (Harding, 1986). The goal of liberal feminist research is therefore to add the category of "women" to that of "men" (Lorber, 1993) to construct balanced objective science. Harding, however, argues that there is no single "woman's perspective" and that there are problems with simply adding women to the research design. Liberal feminism has thus been said to be a compromise that is unworkable (MacKinnon, 1987).

Constructing an equal, opposite "woman's perspective" using the methods of empirical analytic science produces normalized truth that does not simply describe differences. Instead, it perpetuates the marginalized status of women by giving the power associated with social science explanations to existing stereotypical notions, thus strengthening them. Marital arguments, as a result of the findings of social science, can now be filled with new epithets. Instead of calling each other "lazy, good-for-nothing bastard" and "conniving bitch," we have research to support the practice of calling each other "violence-addicted bastard" and "co-dependent bitch."

Feminist standpoint theory attempts to construct knowledge from the perspective of the lives of individual women using qualitative (also called interpretive) research methods. Feminist standpoint epistemology argues that women should use their own research methods because the methods are different from those of men. There are problems with this kind of essentializing epistemology as well. Adding different methods to the masculine research arsenal has the same problems as simply adding women to the sampling frame. The characterization of interpretive methods as methods women use assures that men will avoid using them.

Feminist postmodernist epistemology argues that science creates reality instead of mirroring reality. Feminist postmodernist epistemology does not, however, accept the notion that all explanations have the same social value and argues that some knowledge creations can be preferable to others, within a specific context. According to postmodern feminists, it is important to ask whose interests are being promoted by each of the various possible interpretations that can be made by using different research traditions. Feminist postmodernist epistemology is suspicious of the empirical analytic assumptions inherent in any science, quantitative or qualitative (Harding, 1986).

Marks (1995), however, sounds a cautionary note:

> . . . feminist discourses are legitimately fearful of universalizing language, but these discourses run the risk of ignoring theories that are suspicious of progress and social change, theories that attempt to come to terms with human situations and questions for which there are neither practical solutions nor logical answers (Marks, 1995, p. 286).

Traynor (1997), however, agrees with Lather (1991) that emancipatory research need not be stultified into inaction by the sheer difficulty of critiquing essentializing discourse while at the same time not presuming to speak absolute truth.

There may never be one single feminist epistemology (Alcoff & Potter, 1993). Riger (1992), for example, claims that all forms of feminist epistemology are useful and argues against the existence of one feminist method. There is some agreement that feminist research should not only be about women but also for women, helping to change the world as well as describe it. Riger points out, however, that this agreement can become another authoritarian view, granting privilege to the researcher in yet another way, by ascribing false consciousness to the subjects. She contends that feminism is most useful as a set of questions that challenge the prevailing asymmetries of power and androcentric assumptions in science and society rather than as a basis for a unique method (Riger, 1992, p. 737). What postmodern feminism has accomplished is to shatter the view that science is impersonal and acontextual. Conversely, we need not assume that the scientific method should be all context without sub-stance (Riger, 1992).

Harding (1986) also argues against the existence of any strictly feminist methodology but also claims that the empirical analytic method is inherently flawed. Men's and women's experiences are not simply equally plausible explanations for a knowable separate reality. Women's view as equally legitimate to men's is a relativism that feminists such as Harding reject. Harding argues that feminism rejects the androcentric bias of the male view and is therefore a preferable choice (Harding, 1986). "Members of an oppressed group are more likely than are their oppressors to be suspicious of false claims made about the oppressed group" (Harding, 1991, p. 41).

> One key to success in knowledge development with diverse populations is to invite marginalized people to talk at length about the health problems they face, the obstacles that block their access to health care and other resources, and what they believe is needed to remedy their situations. While this seems almost too simple to be efficacious, the truth is that it is rarely done in research or practice in any discipline. (Hall, Stevens, & Meleis, 1994, p. 35)

Rejecting bias and oppression are fundamental assumptions of feminist research that are superficially at odds with Foucaultian discourse analysis. Harding (1991) questions the possibility of feminists using male science for the liberatory ends of feminism. Harding (1986) asks, "Is it possible to use for emancipatory ends sciences that are apparently so intimately involved in Western, bourgeois, and masculine projects?" (p. 9). The various feminist epistemologies approach this question differently, according to Harding. Liberal feminist empiricism holds that the problem with empirical analytic science is simply that bad science has been conducted because it did not take into account women's experience. When this situation is rectified, all will be well. According to feminist standpoint epistemology, the problem with science is that it comes from a male standpoint. When we add female methods to science, all will be well. These positions rely on essentialized identities of maleness and femaleness, however. Feminist postmodernism, following Foucault, Nietzsche, Derrida, Rorty, Lacan, and Feyerabend, reject the objective/subjective dichotomy that is an assumption of modern empirical analytic science and, instead, analyze on the basis of local descriptions of power politics.

Foucault refused to characterize any perspective or position as better or less oppressive than any other, saying that changing power relations is merely a realignment of the lines of force without any objective position from which to judge improvement. Some feminists agree, and some feminists argue that in a specific social context, the direction and manner of reducing oppression may be perfectly clear, justifiable, and preferable.

Some feminists hold that qualitative or interpretive research is the only real feminist research. Others argue that using multiple methods is more feminist. Bleier (1984) argues that feminists must expose dualisms and dichotomies and not reject any method out of hand. A feminist interpretation is just that—another interpretation. Feminist deconstruction of authoritative voice and power is only one more interpretation (Sapiro, 1995, p. 304). "Feminists have to accept that there is no technique of analysis or methodological logic that can neutralize the social nature of interpretation" (Maynard & Purvis, 1994, p. 7). The factors that "contribute to various strategies of interpretation" need to be made explicit (Maynard & Purvis, 1994, p. 7).

Burnard (1995), on the other hand, argues that it is completely artificial for researchers to "analyze" qualitative data looking for meaning. "Qualitative analysis is always post-hoc" (Burnard, 1995, p. 58). Words are used in so many ways and context is so important that we cannot really ever "get it." "What really happened has been lost" (p. 61). For this reason, feminists often go back to the subjects and check on their interpretations with them before they publish. It is Burnard's opinion, however, that further refinements in qualitative technologies, such as better video or computer software that can capture mood, will solve the problems with determining the true meaning. It seems questionable, however, that purely technological advances will erase the philosophical and political problem of interpretation.

Consider the interpretive research of Belenky, Clinchy, Goldberger, and Tarule (1986), *Women's Ways of Knowing*. Crawford (1989), using Harding's (1986) discussion of feminist epistemologies as described previously, has addressed the problem of interpretation in this research. Crawford argues that first, the work is bad science. The book attempts to compare a completely separate population of females to what has been published about males. Second, the work is a kind of phenomenology, purporting to examine the lived experience of women, and yet the authors continually compare their interpretations to studies of men. Because our society is so androcentric, "psychological research that demonstrates sex differences is likely to be interpreted as demonstrating new sources of biological deficiency in women" (Crawford, 1989, p. 138). The language then becomes universalized and essentialized and all women are assumed to fit the research. Any man who finds parts of this work that apply to himself would disavow any resemblance to his own behavior. One of the worthy goals of feminism, according to Harding (1991), is to further a more complex understanding of *why* western science has felt such a need to create a whole succession of essentialized others such as women, nature, other-than-White races, and so on.

Now consider the interpretive research of Benner (1984) concerning novice and expert behavior in nurses. Cash (1995) has presented a critique of Benner's interpretation of nursing expertise. While purporting to describe nursing expert *behavior* in context based on the Dreyfus (1982) model of situational understanding, Benner instead describes expert *nurses*, based on the judgment of authority and tradition by using experienced evaluators from the same nursing unit. Cash argues that Benner ignores issues of power in clinical practice, resulting not in the empowerment of clinical nursing but in the establishment of clinical salary ladders by which the hospital bureaucracy can differentially reward obedience to policy and procedure.

Feminist research analyzes situations and behavior on the basis of an interpretation of the power relations that function within that environment. Feminist research assumes that gender is a relationship, not a thing, and that gender is defined by the relations between people that are much more varied than is generally assumed in empirical analytic science (Harding, 1991). This assumption is similar to the postmodern assumption by Foucault that power is not a thing; it is a relationship that creates a web of influence relations.

Riger advocates an "interactional" view of gender, which assumes that there is a preexisting component and a social component to gender that interact continuously within a context (Riger, 1992). Hubbard (1990) goes further, arguing that the very idea that genes cause things is inappropriately reductionist and that context has been greatly undervalued and ignored. Empirical analytic science has consistently failed to take into account social context (Cowan, 1994). Barbara McClintock is the exception here, calling attention to context as well as a reductionist particle in her work with the genetics of corn. She has shown that genes alone do not cause traits and that instead the process is more complicated and involves context, translocation, and other influences from the environment (Keller, 1983).

DISCOURSE ANALYSIS AS A POSTMODERN FEMINIST METHODOLOGY

Modernism is defined as "a school of thought which posits that reason is the source of progress and that the increasing development of science and its associated technologies are a benign, indeed desirable, influence in society" (Cheek & Gibson, 1996, p. 84). There is no single unified postmodern position except that all variants share "a critique and challenge [to] the theoretical discourse of the modern" (p. 84). Postmodernist philosophers have criticized empirical analytic science from the marginalized standpoint, problematizing the ideology of dominant science (Traynor, 1997).

A method is a technique for gathering evidence, while a methodology is a theory of how research should proceed (Harding, 1986, p. 2). Postmodern feminist methodologies include discourse analysis. Discourse analysis is a postmodern methodology of analyzing text, as defined in the broadest sense, for the purpose of interpreting the existing power relations. Analyzing discourse for the purpose of discovering whose interests are being served is a form of social criticism with a long history in the discipline of linguistics that has only recently been applied by postmodernists to social relations. Discourse analysis does not claim to be value neutral. The success of discourse analysis depends on the analyst's ability to provide logical arguments instead of comparison against static criteria for truth (Alcoff & Potter, 1993, p. 736). The same could be said of any philosophical argument, but the application to scientific discourses is relatively new. " . . . combining postmodern theories and emancipatory practices will help us to see more clearly the organizational structures and the social processes that reproduce medical dominance and nursing submission" (Fahy, 1997, p. 27).

Discourse analysis focuses on the social features, political ramifications, and power relations inherent in textual and behavioral aspects of a body of knowledge. Discourses objectify and construct people as subjects for research within the discipline. In other words, subjects are "spoken into existence by the available discourses" in both inclusionary and exclusionary ways (Van Der Riet, 1995, p. 149). This powerful process of power/knowledge used by well established discourses serves to silence and marginalize resistance to the normal that has been constructed and reinforced by the discourse. Discourses frame thought, speech, and action by encouraging some ways of talking and knowing and by discouraging others. What is said is as important as what is not said. Discourse analysis "illuminates the metaphors inherent in language, confronts the politics of language, shows what has become normalized truth and, as a result, highlights the unchallenged authoritative presuppositions . . . " (Eade & Bradshaw, 1995, p. 61).

Discourse analysis consists of "a number of different approaches to language" (Harper, 1995, p. 347). The use of language is a social action. People say what they do in order to serve specific interests and this may or may not be intentional. Discourse, including scientific discourse, is never value neutral. Instead, discourse unintentionally perpetuates certain power/knowledge arrangements to the exclusion of others. Reality is therefore socially constructed by many different interacting discourses. Social power/knowledge is not something a person possesses, but something that groups of people perform together. (Harper, 1995, p. 348).

Harper (1989), following Hollway (1989), notes that "the theoretical goal of any discourse analysis is not to ensure the methodological conditions for discovery of truth (e.g. through the perfection of sampling) but to understand the conditions under which differing accounts are produced and how meaning is assumed to be produced from them." (Harper, 1995, p. 350).

Discourse analysis can make sense of contradictory data that would be uninterpretable on an objective measurement scale by identifying different discourses that apply to the same passage. Not only does the personal conscious interest of the speaker with respect to the interviewer need to be considered but also the unconscious participation of the speaker in established dominant discourses. Freedom to position oneself among competing disciplines is a strong indication of power (Harper, 1995, p. 352).

The first feminist research was grounded in what was called *women's experience*, a radical concept at the time. Subsequently, however, it has been charged that "women's experience" has become a reified category, becoming an end in itself, analogous to the unimpeachable evidence of the empirical data of male science. Darbyshire (Emden, 1997) points out that there should be no privilege of voices as data and no archetypal authentic voice to which to appeal when addressing conflicting claims. It can be argued that marginalized groups have committed the same errors as dominant groups by offering universal explanations for various forms of oppression and by "privileging the experience of the oppressed" (Traynor, 1997, p. 99).

Qualitative research can become the new orthodoxy, as restrictive as the old one (Darbyshire, 1997). The critique of objectivity in social theory and some feminisms has been shown to be as universalizing as any other. "Knowledge always carries an implicit domination and power over the known. . . . The authority associated with the unique insight of any particular group is . . . no longer credible (Traynor, 1997, p. 100). This insight can, however, cause paralysis in any dedicated emancipatory project due to the fear of privileging some voices over others. "However, emancipation itself can be understood as an Enlightenment project with ever-present possibilities for domination" (Traynor, 1997, p. 100). The process of exposing domination and oppression can be construed as constructing a new boss, the same as the old boss.

Postmodernism has therefore been called nihilistic linguistic games and poor scholarship offering no standards for the choosing of one policy over another (Zbilut, 1997) and a "hoax" (Kermode & Brown, 1996). Traynor (1997), on the contrary, argues that postmodernism asserts the basis for choosing is contextual instead of universal. In views based solely on power, structural inequalities are ignored, but Traynor argues that Foucault's work on power demonstrates the multiplicity of power without dismissing the importance of the study of structural inequalities. Such an insight can "give sophistication to transformative work" (Traynor, 1997, p. 102).

Transformative work then can be understood as challenging a totalizing narrative without setting up universal standards for evaluation or knowledge generation. Fahy (1997) argues that "Postmodern notions of power and subjectivity can strengthen the theoretical power of emancipatory studies" (p. 32).

Traynor also cautions against too optimistic a view that postmodernism can provide the basis for dialogue between groups of people based on discursive commonalities. Following Parsons (1995), he emphasizes the crucial dilemmas of legitimation and representation for current nursing research (also see Denzin, 1997). If ideology produces language, then there is no "authentic" language for understanding the world and no privileging of subjects' voices in identifying the oppressed. Indeed, the "voices" of marginalized people have been said to mix the discourse of the dominant discourses of their context and their own discourse, in a conscious attempt to seem more acceptable to dominant groups (Hall, Stevens, & Meleis, 1994). Strategies adopted by researchers to avoid this dilemma have included using multiple voices in the research, presenting the research findings to the subjects for their approval, and including the researcher as another voice in the research. This latter assumes that the researcher is "just another voice" to be added, when it seems clear that the researcher is in a much more influential and powerful position than just another voice. It is much more likely that one or at most a few voices that belong to the authors will predominate (Walker, 1997).

HOW FEMINISM HAS ADAPTED FOUCAULTIAN DISCOURSE ANALYSIS

The feminist process variables, or process criteria, are discursive modifications of Habermas' (1984) notion of a communicative ideal. Habermas (1984) argued that the communicative ideal of rationality is approached by two goals for the process of discourse: autonomy and responsibility. Habermas defines autonomy as the ability and willingness to participate openly in conversation, saying that it requires understanding one's own values, interests, and needs. Responsibility means ensuring all participants can function autonomously in the conversation by paying attention to group dynamics, knowledge imbalances, and power differences. Rationality, for Habermas, is influenced by the confidence one can have in the outcome of the conversation and is approached by working toward these two communicative ideals.

Some feminists have revised Habermas' notions of ideal speech situations and their relation to communicative rationality. These feminists have noted that Habermas' notion rests on a transcendental individualistic model and abstract notions of fairness, justice, and reciprocity as normatively achievable goals (Calhoun, 1992). Habermas does not consider whether an acceptable form of rationality might begin with relationships rather than individual persons. The very notion of individual is demonstrated by postmodernists to be historically and culturally specific. If the starting point for discourse becomes relationships instead of individuals, then one must necessarily take into account the nonequivalence and noninterchangeability of persons—that is, their situatedness. Diversity of situations is thus seen as desirable in feminist methodology.

Fraser (1989), for example, critiques Habermas' communicative ideal from the postmodern standpoint of power relations, hegemony, and patriarchal society. The determination of a person's right to speak within a discourse is a socially constructed act and an interested move of power. For Habermas, communicative consensus assures the autonomy and responsibility of speakers in truth claims within ideal speech situations. This consensus is a communicative ideal and is not found in real human situations. The pursuit of an ideal speech situation can become a rhetorical exercise that is as oppressive as the one it seeks to replace, unless it examines its own interests, processes, and goals.

Fraser argues that Habermas' criteria for rational discourse ignores women's oppressed group status (Fraser, 1989). The goal of communicative consensus assumes that individuals are capable of helping each other to see clearly and working equally toward consensus. Being embedded in a network of power/knowledge limits individuals' capacity to reason with clarity. Participants are further limited in their actions due to the possible consequences in their lives. This is to say that individuals are not all equally free to choose. The definition of an individual with certain rights, who has the potential to become a speaker in Habermas' account, is based on invested power positions. According to Fraser, Habermas' concepts are transcendental and not located in situated bodies.

Some feminists therefore add to Habermas' communicative goals of autonomy and responsibility the notions of the connectedness among participants, intersubjectivity, situatedness, and the roles of emotion, diversity, and intuition as supportive of group rationality. Allen (1992), for example, explicates these process variables with respect to nursing inquiry. The notion of situatedness suggests that interaction focus first on values, perspectives, and worldviews. After exploring the situatedness of the participants, it would be appropriate to move on to the issue at hand. These foci are not seen as a form a relativism but as a part of the process wherein speakers explicate their worldview and perspective instead of forcing people to guess about it, enabling them to assess how much they share with each other (Allen, 1992). Process ideals do not guarantee rational outcomes. Instead, work on process simply highlights the power and context issues that Habermas ignored, in order to avoid co-optation of resistance (Allen, 1992, p. 13).

The feminist process criteria represent an historical shift away from speakers and authors writing for themselves and then applying their conclusions to other groups. One implication of this approach is that in order to assess the rationality of the discourse, the existence of an ongoing reconciled intersubjectivity among the community of speakers must be evaluated (Allen, 1992).

Consequently, when faced with competing claims, feminists analyze the data and the context in which the claim arose in order to provide evidence with respect to whether or not the process respected autonomy, responsibility, situatedness, interconnectedness, diversity, emotion, and intuition.

POSTMODERN FEMINIST DISCOURSE ANALYSIS IN NURSING RESEARCH

Nursing has historically been uncritical of biomedical discourse (Eade & Bradshaw, 1995, p. 61). Biomedical discourse, following empirical analytic science, assumes that the world can be divided into subjective and objective information and that only the objective is useful to science, medicine, and health. Furthermore, the subjective is often linked with the feminine by using such words as *irrational, emotional,* and *soft science* (Eade & Bradshaw, 1995, p. 62). "Discourse analysis is valuable as a way of understanding alternative views of nursing knowledge" (Heartfield, 1996, p. 100). Hall, Stevens, & Meleis (1994) argued that "As a practice discipline, nursing requires means of inquiry that are durable and flexible enough to be applied in circumstances where statistical measures are unwieldy, too sweeping in their generalizations, nonspecific to the question at hand, or too economically burdensome in their requirements" (1994, p. 24).

Discourse analysis based on Foucaultian power analysis has been suggested for nursing research (Powers, 1996). Cheek & Porter (1997) describe some strengths and weaknesses of Foucaultian theory of power for use in nursing research. Cheek lists the strengths as a focus on discourse, recognition of power/knowledge, descriptions of disciplinary techniques and their unintended consequences, the notion of the body as constructed by competing discourses, the identification of the clinical gaze, and the suggestion that resistance is possible. Porter lists the limitations as rejection of possible emancipatory projects as one more totalizing narrative, problematizing the 'authentic' voice, the relativism of truth claims, the dismissal of the subject, and the difficulty of using a Foucaultian perspective to produce alternatives. Cheek answers that researchers need to let go of the notion that there has to be certain knowledge of anything, that problematizing the authentic voice can be a good thing to do, and that analyzing the contextualized effects of power need not produce a grand narrative. Despite differences of opinion, Foucaultian discourse analyses continue to be produced.

As a practice discipline, nursing embraces a practical, problem-solving element. Situational context-based problem solving has long held lower social status than scientific knowledge generation. For example, Peerson (1995) points out that Foucault neglected to document the social distinction of medicine and surgery in his archaeology of the birth of the clinic. Surgery was more intent on solving practical problems and not on the production of medical knowledge (p. 110). Medicine, after it enfolded surgery in an imperialistic expansion, configured its gaze to ignore social conditions and subjective statements in favor of empirical analytic research aimed at constructing a hierarchy of diagnoses and treatments. Due to the power of empirical analytic knowledge production and control, there are no social controls over the limits of the medical gaze (Peerson, 1995, p. 112). Substituting methadone for heroin, for example, is considered "better" because it affords medical control instead of leaving control to the individual addict. Assigning "vulnerability" status by assessing relative risk is an extremely powerful social move of power (Hall et al., 1994).

The discipline of nursing seeks to develop this same power base for itself. Consequently, the discipline of nursing is acutely aware of its lower social status and continually strives for some unique scientific method or subject that can generate unique nursing knowledge using empirical analytic science. Traynor (1996) argues in this context that nursing discourse has continually reshaped its own definition in order to develop power and professional status in a manner that reflected the current powerful language of the day, whether it is caring, science, cost-benefit, or economic rationalism.

Furthermore, nursing discourse reflects the competing views of the different feminist epistemologies without widely acknowledging the more generalized abstract debate.

May and Purkis (1995), support the idea that Foucault's work can be used as a method for advancing critical understandings of the *effects* of nursing practice which are rarely addressed in interpretive studies. These authors argue that nursing discourse has undertaken to recast ordinary features of daily life into nursing problems, thus participating in the medicalization (or nursification) of social control. "The idea that everyday life is intrinsically morbid appears to underpin diagnostic categories" (May and Purkis, 1995, p. 286). Nursing has constructed itself as a discipline of human relations instead of as a technical practice concerned with physiological functions. For example, the nurse-patient relationship is commonly taught as a therapeutic tool for nurses, but what does it really do? In order for the relationship to be therapeutic, the patient must be discursively constructed as the recipient of nursing care (May & Purkis, 1995), a malleable object of the discursive strategies of the therapeutic relationship as defined by nursing discourse. Nurses are thus expected to change patients by sheer force of personality.

No one discusses nursing as manual labor on a human body because of the current social shift in view of the patient from an object/body to an experiencing subject that is the object of nursing *care* (for which, read "control"). Nursing is a set of practices located within an organizational context, but nursing has shifted from vocational rhetoric to rhetoric that demands professional status. The long term effect of this shift on patients has not yet been examined, and the effect may not be positive. A discourse analysis of these effects would ask the following question: In whose interest is the discursive construction of the whole patient as the object of nursing care?

Traynor (1996) argues that the last 30 years of nursing theory have in some ways not affected practice at all and in other ways have seriously affected nursing practice. The entire body of nursing theory has been constructed to underpin the project of the professionalization of nursing. Nurses are being taught how to discipline patients into systematic expositions that satisfy the nurse and give the nurse acceptable reasons for doing the tasks of nursing. The only way a patient can retain privacy in this situation is not to talk at all. The moral component of nursing has been buried under a set of prescribed research-based tasks that pathologize everyday life.

The discourse of professionalism in nursing continues. Huntington, Gilmour, and O'Connell (1996) argue that nursing is colonized by other disciplines and until we have our own unique scientific knowledge, we will not be a profession. Caring is still suggested as the {female} essence and future of nursing (Gordon, 1991).

Kermode (1995) uses "critical discourse analysis," which he defines, following Fairclough (1992), as showing "how discourse is shaped by relations of power and ideologies, and the constructive effects discourse has upon social identities, social relations and systems of knowledge or belief" (Kermode,

1995, p. 9). He analyzes the professionalism discourse in nursing and finds it to be supportive of the status quo, consistent with the consolidation of power in fewer and fewer hands, and elitist with respect to race and education (Kermode, 1995, p. 10). Traynor (1997) agrees, pointing out that professionals discursively create their clients in order that their discipline can deal with them. In subscribing to the discourse of professionalism, nurses therefore reinforce their own oppression. He quotes Ivan Illich (1973) regarding the term *professional imperialism*, which includes the concept of professional turf. All professions defend and seek to expand their turf into areas held by other professions.

The unintended consequences of the project of science-based professionalism are visible in many concepts supported by nursing research, such as empowerment, caring, health promotion, and holism. Traynor (1997) argues, for example, that the discourse of empowerment in nursing professionalism has necessarily become misconstrued to reflect an act done by one person to another. Nursing has embraced this concept and changed it so as to reinforce nursing's power over clients, instead of the self-liberation of clients by clients. This inevitably oppresses both nurses and patients and sets up both the nurse and the patient for failure.

The discourse of caring has become so pervasive and prescriptive that it promotes caring in nurses to the point of co-dependency, a trait that has become essentialized to the definition of women. The tyranny of the discourse of caring has become yet another authority. There is no room in the caring discourse for critique—you are either a caring nurse or you are not, and if you are not, then you are clearly a failure as a nurse (Traynor, 1997).

The discourse of health promotion focuses the nurse's attention on the individual patient and blames the victim for ill health and "unhealthy" lifestyles. There is no room in the discourse of health promotion for structural problems of unemployment and oppression or the problem of race as a social instead of a genetic category (Kaufman & Cooper, 1995). The nursing discourse of health promotion ignores social causes of ill health. Instead, it focuses on helping individuals cope with a bad context instead of including the patient in a radical critique of the social context. Nursing students are taught the proper ways to interact with a stereotypical "Black person" or "Asian person" without letting the patient determine the structure and process of the clinical encounter. Furthermore, the health promotion movement causes people to feel guilty for their own sickness because it is a moral failure not to obey good advice. The only way people can keep their own individuality is by defying good advice and participating in dangerous or unhealthy lifestyles, preferring risk to anonymity. Quoting Illich (1977), Peerson (1995) states that "health professions . . . destroy the potential of people to deal with their human weakness, vulnerability and uniqueness in a personal and autonomous way" (Peerson, 1995, p. 33).

The theory of holism (or wholism) is another oppressive technology wielded by nurses at the expense of patients' autonomy. The discipline of nursing seeks the morally high ground of treating the "whole patient" whether or not patients want them to do so. Despite the ethical overtones, holism is a move of power and control in the name of professionalism. The discourse of holism is another ideology that has the effect of silencing critique. Nurses, in attempting to treat the whole person, create a speaking subject that can more easily be controlled (Peerson, 1995) by requiring the patients to confess their innermost secrets and habits to the nurse. Only by refusing to talk can patients retain their privacy. These patients are then labeled noncompliant.

In psychiatric nursing, for example, confession is assumed to be liberating for the client, but what the clients are supposed to confess is predetermined by the nursing literature. The nurse works diligently to obtain the proper information from the client to fit one diagnosis or another. The act of confession becomes a technique of control (Bleier, 1984) despite the assertion that the nurse "shares" power with the patient in the psychotherapeutic relationship (Price and Mullarkey, 1996). Nurses elicit confessions that are the data used to assign scientifically determined categories of pathology. Clearly, these social moves of power are performed with good intentions, with the "good of the client" in mind. However, the definition of the "good of the client" or "successful therapy" are also based on knowledge development by nursing research with respect to normality and not on what an individual client wants.

Harper (1995) argues that discourse analysis can be useful in research on mental health in several ways. It can focus on process instead of outcome. It can locate therapy positions in wider social discourses. It can deconstruct the process of diagnosis, showing its social complexities instead of assuming a simple scientific process of categorization. In the discourse on mental health and illness, a discourse analysis would not be explanatory (for example, "She is doing that because she is depressed") but would open up questions to be explored, such as "what interests are served by the concept of 'depression' in this context?" (Harper, 1995, p. 348). Harper argues for three directions for future work. First, the analyses should "embrace diversity." Secondly, mental health services should represent this diversity. Third, mental health practitioners should "explore therapeutic alternatives" that are nonpathologizing (Harper, 1995, p. 354).

Without a thorough analysis of the power relations within the practice of nursing, social change cannot be accomplished. Discourse analysis is a promising methodology for nursing inquiry. "Only in a society fully committed to educational equity can we develop research programs that focus on the learning and teaching process rather than on the possibility of inherent racial or sexual deficiencies" (Fausto-Sterling, 1985, p. 222).

Traynor (1997) summarizes the crucial questions facing the discourse analyst in nursing research. He does this by questioning the authority of his own analysis, saying that he does not privilege one discourse over the other. He addressed the question of the identification of an oppressed group by refusing to identify anyone as an oppressed group. These commitments resulted in the following assumptions in his work:

1. Inquiry can be characterized as a recontextualizing of beliefs.
2. Explanation is another interpretation and has no more rational basis than any other.
3. Totalizing narratives have an inhibiting effect.
4. There is a danger in exchanging one discursive identity for another because it can create new oppressions.
5. Critique uses the same persuasive techniques as the works it attempts to critique; yet critique insists on its own rigor and structure and is not arbitrary.
6. Any truth claims produced must be understood as contextual.

Traynor therefore describes his work not as an emancipatory project but as "causing trouble" for those who are at that moment having their version of truth and rationality dominate others' versions (Traynor, 1997, p. 106).

EXAMPLES OF DISCOURSE ANALYSIS IN NURSING INQUIRY

Eade and Bradshaw (1995) have performed a discourse analysis that attempts to deconstruct and analyze the discourse concerning the "worried well." The authors defined the *worried well* as those women who seek medical attention but do not have a medical diagnosis and are perceived by medical practitioners as wasting medical resources. Often a psychiatric diagnosis is assigned by medicine so that at least something concrete can be done. Women have been characterized as more susceptible to mental illness by nature, and unhappiness in a woman is therefore perceived as a result of her femaleness. Something about being a woman makes all women at risk for depression. Since no definitive biological answers have been generated, the condition is medicalized and treated with drugs, most often antidepressants.

Unhappy women are considered to be emotionally sick, but unhappy men are counseled with respect to solving their problems. Men also become depressed, but the condition is not diagnosed as such (Tavris, 1992). Eade and Bradshaw conclude that nursing should continue to deconstruct biomedical discourse. However, by limiting their discourse to women because they "are more likely to be categorized as worried well" (Eade & Bradshaw, 1995, p. 62), these authors have committed a similar error as those they wish to critique, by providing a normalizing discourse for unhappy women and marginalizing the discourse on men who display these same characteristics of the worried well.

Van Der Riet (1995) analyzed the discourse of students learning how to massage patients by massaging each other. She concludes that learning and performing massage is more difficult for male students than female students because of the sexual aspects of massage. The students prefer to call it a backrub instead of massage so that it is more clinical sounding. Van Der Riet recommends recognition of possible gender differences and the sexual nature of massage itself in the teaching of clinical techniques.

Cheek and Gibson (1996) have analyzed the discourse of nursing administration of medications. They found the dominant discourses in the text to be science and law. Discourses that involve the patient and the nurse as human beings and discourses of resistance to policy and procedure are absent. The authors challenge nurses to develop positions that are capable of generating resistance strategies to blind adherence to policy and procedure at the expense of contextualized understanding.

Breda and colleagues (1997) claim to have increased the autonomy of nurses in a small rural psychiatric hospital by using participatory action research (PAR), which is a form of discourse analysis (or critical ethnography) that involves the subjects in the analysis during the research process (see Kemmis & McTaggert, 2000). Breda and colleagues defined *autonomy* as the freedom to act on what one knows. They proposed to develop a critical consciousness in the nurses in this facility. Following Reason (1994), they said there were two objectives of PAR: "1) to produce knowledge and action directly useful to a group of people—through research, adult education and sociopolitical action and 2) to empower people at a second, deeper level through the process of constructing and using their own knowledge" (p. 324).

The aim of the study was to produce autonomous knowledge and action over one year. During nursing retreats, nurses discussed their lack of autonomy and concluded that they were an oppressed group. A study group was formed, and the members identified strengths and weaknesses in their knowledge base. When trying to put new knowledge into action, members were able to identify barriers to successful implementation of new ideas. They increased their involvement with treatment teams and client conferences. Hospital authorities and physicians reported that they were impressed, and nurses felt more like they were acting on their own knowledge. The themes identified by the nurses were ownership of practice, emphasis on wellness and healing, and clients as partners. The authors concluded that nurses can successfully challenge institutional norms. The nurses felt as though they were beginning to transform oppressive practices.

It could be argued, however, that the nurses simply became better at being good institutional nurses. If they had really challenged the norms of the bureaucratic order, they would have been chastised or disciplined. Instead, the authorities were impressed. Their work could not have represented any real threat to the institutional norms because there would have been resistance to their efforts. They may have raised their own consciousness about participating more fully within their limited options, but they did not expand their options or raise the consciousness of anybody else.

Lupton (1994) performed a discourse analysis of the discourse on AIDS in the Australian print press in 1987. She identified the metaphors that the press used for condoms, both positive and negative. She concluded that condoms, having been linked to AIDS by both positive and negative metaphors in the press, have not become more popular despite the knowledge that they reduce the spread of HIV. Lupton concludes that condoms will not become acceptable unless the public discourse changes.

Ainsworth-Vaughn (1995) analyzed the discourse between patients and oncologists in a specialty clinic setting. She described the discursive strategies that were used for gaining power within the encounter: interruptions, questions, the invocation of structural affiliation, and topic control. She concluded that the physician's interpretation became dominant over the patient's interpretation of the situation.

Heartfield (1996) performed a discourse analysis of nursing documentation. She concluded that the written documentation of nursing practice was more heavily influenced by dominant discourses of medicine and science than the oral knowledge of nursing practice. She analyzed the nurses' written documentation in six complete patient records. She describes the discursive properties of the text, saying that they included an emphasis on the dominant voice of physicians and the absence of patients' voices. She argues that the text constructs an objective "patient" out of a private "person" by focusing on body parts and deficits. She found no evidence for a holistic view of the object of nursing care, the patient.

Heartfield noted that the key factor that orders the entire hospital contractual arrangement is a medical diagnosis. Nursing care is therefore an indirect and hidden part of this contract, functioning to translate a human experience into objective bits of medically interpretable, and therefore useful, data. Heartfield argues that being able to function as a translator affords nurses power within biomedicine and at the same time allows nurses to perform other functions that are not recorded because they are not valued. This invisible nursing work is a discourse of resistance that creates space for the unacknowledged work of nursing. Existing power arrangements are therefore supported while maintaining space for practices of resistance.

These examples of discourse analysis in nursing inquiry represent a developing interest in questions of power, methodology, gender, oppression, science, and the nature of knowledge in nursing practice. As more graduate nursing students study a wider variety of research methods, we may expect more discourse analyses to be performed and published in the coming years.

REFERENCES

Ainsworth-Vaughn, N. (1995). Claiming power in the medical encounter: The whirlpool discourse. *Qualitative Health Research*, 5(3), 270–291.

Alcoff, L., & Potter, E. (1993). *Feminist epistemologies*. New York: Routledge.

Allen, D. G. (1992). Feminism, relativism and the philosophy of science: An overview. In J. L. Thompson, D. G. Allen and L. Rodrigues-Fisher (Eds.), *Critique, Resistance and Action: Working Papers in the Politics of Nursing*. New York: NLN.

Belenky, M. F., Clinchy, B. M., Goldberger, N. R., & Tarule, J. M. (1986). *Women's ways of knowing: The development of self, voice, and mind*. New York: Basic Books.

Benner, P. (1984). *From novice to expert: Excellence and power in clinical nursing practice*. Menlo Park, CA: Addison Wesley.

Blackwood, E. (1993). Sexuality and gender in certain native American tribes: The case of cross-gender females. In L. Richardson & V. Taylor (Eds.), *Feminist frontiers III* (pp. 140–150). New York: McGraw-Hill.

Bleier, R. (1984). *Science and gender: A critique of biology and its theories on women*. New York: Pergamon.

Breda, K. L., Anderson, M. A., Hansen, L., Hayes, D., Pillion, C., & Lyon, P. (1997). Enhanced nursing autonomy through participatory action research. *Nursing Outlook, 45*(2), 76–81.

Burnard, P. (1995). Unspoken meanings: qualitative research and multi-media analysis. *Nurse Researcher, 3*(1), 55–64.

Calhoun, C. (1992). Culture, history and the problem of specificity in social theory. In S. Seidman and D. Wagner (Eds.), *Postmodernism and Social Theory*. Cambridge, MA: Blackwell.

Cancian, F. M. (1993). The feminization of love. In L. Richardson & V. Taylor (Eds.), *Feminist frontiers III* (pp. 292–301). New York: McGraw-Hill.

Cash, K. (1995). Benner and expertise in nursing: A critique. *International Journal of Nursing Studies, 32*(6), 527–534.

Cheek, J., & Gibson, T. (1996). The discursive construction of the role of the nurse in medication administration: An exploration of the literature. *Nursing Inquiry, 3*(2), 83–90.

Cheek, J., & Porter, S. (1997). Reviewing Foucault: Possibilities and problems for nursing and health care. *Nursing Inquiry, 4*(2), 108–119.

Cowan, S. (1994). Community attitudes towards people with mental health problems: A discourse analytic approach. *Journal of Psychiatric and Mental Health Nursing, 1*, 15–22.

Crawford, M. (1989). Feminist epistemologies and women's ways of knowing. In M. Crawford & M. Gentry, *Gender and thought: Psychological perspectives* (pp. 128–145). New York: Springer-Verlag.

Darbyshire, P. (1997). Qualitative research: Is it becoming the new orthodoxy? Editorial, *Nursing Inquiry, 4*(1), 1–2.

Denzin, N. K. (1997). *Interpretive ethnography: Ethnographic practices of the 21st century*. Thousand Oaks, CA: Sage

Dreyfus, S. E. (1982). Formal models vs. human situational understanding. *Office Technol. People, 1*, 133–165.

Eade, G., & Bradshaw, J. (1995). Understanding discourses of the worried well. *Australian and New Zealand Journal of Mental Health Nursing, 4*, 61–69.

Emden, C. (1997). A conversation with Margarete Sandelowski and Philip Darbyshire: Issues in qualitative inquiry. *Nursing Inquiry, 4*(2), 138–141.

Fairclough, N. (1992). *Discourse and social change*. Cambridge: Polity Press.

Fausto-Sterling, A. (1985). *Myths of gender: Biological theories about women and men*. New York: Basic Books.

Fahy, K. (1997). Postmodern feminist emancipatory research: Is it an oxymoron?" *Nursing Inquiry*, 4(1), 27–33.

Ford-Gilboe, N., & Campbell, J. (1996). The mother-headed single-parent family: A feminist critique of the nursing literature. *Nursing Outlook*, 44, 173–83.

Fraser, N. (1989). Unruly Practices: Power, Discourse and Gender in Contemporary Social Theory. Minneapolis: University of Minnesota Press.

Gordon, S. (1991). Fear of caring: The feminist paradox. *American Journal of Nursing*, 91(2), 45–48.

Habermas, J. (1984). *The Theory of Communicative action*. Translated by Thomas McCarthy. Boston: Beacon Press.

Hall, J. M. (1994). The experience of lesbians in Alcoholics Anonymous. *Western Journal of Nursing Research*, 16(5), 556–576.

Hall, J. M., Stevens, P. E., & Meleis, A. I. (1994). Marginalization: A guiding concept for valuing diversity in nursing knowledge development. *Advances in Nursing Science*, 16(4), 23–41.

Harding, S. (1986). *The science question in feminism*. Ithaca: Cornell University Press.

Harding, S. (1991). *Whose science? Whose knowledge?* Ithaca: Cornell University Press.

Harper, D. (1995). Discourse Analysis and 'mental health'. *Journal of Mental Health*, 4, 347–357.

Hartsock, N. (1983). The Feminist Standpoint: Developing the Ground for a Specifically Feminist Historical Materialism. In S. Harding & M. B. Hintikka (Eds.), *Discovering reality: Feminist perspectives on epistemology, metaphysics, methodology, and philosophy of science* (pp. 283–310). Boston: D. Reidel.

Heartfield, M. (1996). Nursing documentation and nursing practice: A discourse analysis. *Journal of Advanced Nursing*, 24, 98–103.

Hollway, W. (1989). *Subjectivity and method in psychology: Gender, meaning and science*. London: Sage.

Hubbard, R. (1990). *The Politics of Women's Biology*. New Brunswick: Rutgers University Press.

Huntington, A., Gilmour, J., & O'Connell, A. (1996). Reforming the practice of nurses: Decolonization or getting out from under. *Journal of Advanced Nursing*, 24, 364–367.

Illich, I. (1973). The professions as a form of imperialism. *New Society*, 13, 633–635.

Illich, I. (1977). *Limits to medicine—Medical nemesis: The expropriation of health*. London: Marion Boyars.

Kaufman, J. S., & Cooper, R. S. (1995). In search of the hypothesis. *Public Health Reports*, 110, 662–667.

Keller, E. F. (1983). *A feeling for the organism: The life and work of Barbara McClintock*. San Francisco: W. H. Freeman.

Kemmis, S., & McTaggart, R. (2000). Participatory action research. In N. K. Denzin & Y. S. Lincoln (Eds.), *Handbook of qualitative research* (2nd Ed.). Thousand Oaks, CA: Sage.

Kermode, S. (1995). Where have all the flowers gone? Nursing's escape from the radical critique. *Contemporary Nurse*, 4, 8–15.

Kermode, S., & Brown, C. (1996). The postmodernist hoax and its effects on nursing. *International Journal of Nursing Studies, 33*(4), 375–384.

Lather, P. (1991). *Getting smart: Feminist research and pedagogy within the postmodern.* London: Routledge.

Lorber, J. (1993). Believing is seeing: Biology as ideology. *Gender & Society, 7*(4), 568–581.

Lupton, D. (1994). The Condom in the age of AIDS: Newly respectable or still a dirty word? A discourse analysis. *Qualitative Health Research, 4*(3), 304 320.

MacKinnon, C. (1987). Feminism, Marxism, method, and the state: Toward feminist jurisprudence. In S. Harding (Ed.), *Feminism and Methodology* (pp. 135–136). Bloomington: Indiana University Press.

Marks, E. (1995). The poetical and the political: The feminist inquiry in French studies. In D. C. Stanton & A. J. Stewart (Eds.), *Feminisms in the academy* (pp. 274–287). Ann Arbor: The University of Michigan Press.

Martin, E. (1991). The egg and the sperm: How science has constructed a romance based on stereotypical male-female roles. *Signs: Journal of Women in Culture and Society, 16*(31), 485–501.

Martin, E. (1997). The new culture of health: Gender and the immune system in America. In M. de Ras & V. Grace (Eds.), *Bodily boundaries, sexualized genders & medical discourses* (pp. 17–26). Palmerston North, New Zealand: Dunmore Press.

May, C. R. & Purkis, M. E. (1995). The configuration of nurse-patient relationships: A critical view. *Scholarly Inquiry for Nursing Practice: An International Journal, 9*(4), 283–295.

Maynard, M., & Purvis, J., Eds. (1994). *Researching women's lives from a feminist perspective.* London: Taylor & Francis.

Parsons, C. (1995). The impact of postmodernism on research methodology: Implications for nursing. *Nursing Inquiry, 2*(1), 22–28.

Peerson, A. (1995). Foucault and modern medicine. *Nursing Inquiry, 2*(3), 106–114.

Powers, P. (1996). Discourse analysis as a methodology for nursing inquiry. *Nursing Inquiry, 3*(4), 207–217.

Price, V., & Mullarkey, K. (1996). Use and misuse of power in the psychotherapeutic relationship. *Mental Health Nursing, 16*(1), 16–17.

Reason, P. (1994). Three approaches to participative inquiry. In N. K. Denzin & Y. S. Lincoln (Eds.), *Handbook of qualitative research* (pp. 324–329). Thousand Oaks, CA: Sage.

Riger, S. (1992). Epistemological debates, feminist voices: Science, social values, and the study of women. *American Psychologist, 47*(6), 730–740.

Sapiro, V. (1995). Feminist studies and political science—and vice versa. In D. C. Stanton & A. J. Stewart (Eds.), *Feminisms in the academy* (pp. 291–310). Ann Arbor: The University of Michigan Press.

Scully, D., & Marolla, J. (1993). Riding the bull at Gilley's: Convicted rapists describe the rewards of rape. In L. Richardson & V. Taylor (Eds.), *Feminist frontiers* III (pp. 402–413). New York: McGraw-Hill.

Stepan, N. L. (1993). Race and gender: The role of analogy in science. In S. Harding (Ed.), *The racial economy of science: Towards a democratic future* (pp. 359–376). Bloomington, IN: Indiana University Press.

Stevens, P. E. (1996). Lesbians and doctors: Experiences of solidarity and domination in health care settings. *Gender & Society*, 10(1), 24–41.

Tavris, C. (1992). *The mismeasure of woman*. New York: Simon and Schuster.

Traynor, M. (1996.) Looking at discourse in a literature review of nursing texts. *Journal of Advanced Nursing*, 23, 1155–1161.

Traynor, M. (1997). Postmodern research: No grounding or privilege, just free-floating trouble making. *Nursing Inquiry*, 4(2), 99–107.

Van Der Riet, P. (1995). Massage and sexuality in nursing. *Nursing Inquiry*, 2(4), 149–156.

Walker, K. (1997). Cutting edges: Deconstructive inquiry and the mission of the border ethnographer. *Nursing Inquiry*, 4(1), 3–13.

Weedon, C. (1987). *Feminist practice & poststructuralist theory*. Oxford: Blackwell.

Worth, H. (1997). Jungle fever: AIDS and the Peter Mwai affair. In M. de Ras & V. Grace (Eds.), *Bodily boundaries, sexualized genders & medical discourses* (pp. 52–65). Palmerston North, New Zealand: Dunmore Press.

Zbilut, J. P. (1997). Joseph Zbilut responds. *Image*, 29(1), 6–7.

CHAPTER 3

PERFORMING A DISCOURSE ANALYSIS

INTRODUCTION

The purpose of this chapter is to describe the process of performing and producing a discourse analysis. The type of discourse analysis described in this chapter is based on the antifoundational perspective of critical theory, Foucault's postmodernist power perspective and feminism. There are similar approaches such as critical hermeneutics, performance ethnography, participatory action research, and critical ethnography, but their descriptions are not included in this book (see Denzin & Lincoln, 2000).

In general, the goal of a discourse analysis is to provide interpretive claims based on a description of power relations in the context of historically specific situations. Discourse analysis is conducted in varying ways depending on the differential emphasis given to the foci of the methodology and the nature of the situated discourse being analyzed. Foucault believed the purpose of discourse analysis is to describe the connections, contradictions, and puzzles of a discourse with the goal of producing a tool for radical political action (Foucault, 1977, p. 205). The emphasis here is that the analysis is a "tool" for radical political action. The analysis, according to Foucault, does not specify the action to be taken by expressing a preference for one outcome over another, or one speaking position over another, as a feminist analysis would.

In order to analyze a discourse, the analyst must read all of it, see it in action, discuss it with people, and read what other people have said about it. The entire body of published work concerning the discourse is usually read with questions such as the ones found later in this chapter in mind. Interviews, if possible, are performed with as many participants as is practical. Observations are performed, if possible, on actions dictated by the discourse. Notes organized under the headings provided by each question are taken during this time. New questions can be formulated and answered. Finally, after all data and notes are reviewed, the claims are generated and written and supported with compilations or quoted data from the discourse itself.

The results are written in philosophical argument style. Context relevant interpretations justified by the analysis are presented and supported. Some discourse analyses are book length, and some are article length, depending on the complexity of the discourse being analyzed. Publication is usually classified as theoretical.

The specific objectives of discourse analysis are (a) to document the historical conditions of the existence of the discourse in genealogy, (b) to describe the socially constructed system of power/knowledge in a structural analysis, and (c) to analyze the effects of the discourse within the web of social power relations in a power analytic. A discourse analysis may combine all three parts into one discussion.

The first part, the genealogy, interprets the historical power influences on the emerging discourse. The second part, the structural discourse analysis, focuses on the internal logical structure of the discourse. The third part, the power analytic, analyzes the power effects related to the functioning of the discourse, including intended and unintended consequences. All three parts are intimately related to each other and are sometimes separated purely for purposes of conceptual clarity (see chapter 4 for an example).

GENEALOGY

The part of a discourse analysis called genealogy, as the name suggests, emphasizes the historical components of the discourse. Genealogy seeks the conditions that made possible the discursive processes practiced in a specific discourse (Kusch, 1991) as the basis for identifying present power relations. "The best way to see that things might be otherwise is to see that they were once otherwise, and in some areas of life, still are" (Dreyfus, 1987, p. 331). Because of the importance of the historical aspect of power relations, genealogy gives priority to analysis of organizing social practices over the analysis of acontextual theory. Accordingly, in *Discipline and Punish: The Birth of the Prison* (1979), Foucault chose to analyze not the history of the *concept of punishment* but the history of the *practice of confinement* that included the analysis of the discourse surrounding the practices (Mish'alani, 1988). Significantly, however, the discourse of prisoners themselves is absent in Foucault's account of the practice of confinement. Feminist practice would advocate adding the voice of the prisoner to that analysis.

Consistent with the postmodern perspective, local narratives with moral intent are preferred by discourse analysts to generalizing theoretical discourse in a genealogy. This is to say that specific contextualized discussions that describe the ethical issues without assuming a position of disinterested inquiry are considered preferable. "Genealogies aim to uncover the social processes concealed by hegemonic essentialist discourses and to implicate these discourses in these formative social process" (Seidman, 1992, p. 70).

From an antifoundational perspective, Foucault did not posit long-term historical continuity and objective meaning to a discourse. Rather, genealogy only assumes that there are historical influences that have had an influence on the regularities of the discourse. The influence of nondiscursive factors is also considered and includes such things as institutions, events, practices, politics, economics, demographics, media, gestures, clothing, style, habits, terminology, and the range of roles to be fulfilled by human subjects (Foss and Gill, 1987).

What a genealogy chooses to look at and the range of material available both reflect its own historical situatedness. A genealogy can show the accidental historical status of the discourse and broaden our perspective to include practices still alive that have not been co-opted or removed (Dreyfus, 1987, p. 331). But doing so does not imply that we can step outside our circumstances or ourselves in a foundational manner and discern, once and for all, what happened and why. Instead, the genealogy widens the view from where the author and/or the readers currently stand to include a broad picture of the historical contribution to the development of the practices of power and resistance in the specific discourse under analysis.

According to Rawlinson (1987), a genealogy is an analysis of the historical emergence of a system of notions and rules for the construction of meaningful statements, justifications, and the concrete material realities and procedures for determining truth and falsity in a discourse (p. 376). The key issue is the historical formation of the authority of the discourse and how it came to have the right to pronounce truth in some region of experience. No assumption is made to the effect that it can be determined exactly how people came to think and talk and act this way in some objective fashion. A genealogy is an interpretation openly arising from a postmodern, antifoundational, feminist orientation concerning the operation of power in a specifically situated context.

In a genealogy, the analyst asks the following questions with respect to the discourse (following Rawlinson, 1987): What other discourses and/or events provided models or ideas that influenced the functioning of the discourse under analysis, and in what ways? What words in the discourse have a linguistic and social history that is significant for assessing the role of the discourse within current power relations? What historical context influenced the development of the discourse? What physical, bodily space was created by being described by the discursive practices of the discourse? What surfaces of emergence and conditions of possibility were acknowledged and appropriated and made visible by this discourse, and by what means? By what processes did the discourse construct the right to pronounce truth in some region of experience? What other discourses were affected and how? What power struggles or turf battles occurred, and what was the outcome? In whose interests was the social construction of this discourse? Whose interests were ignored and/or rejected?

The answers to these questions form the genealogy. On the basis of the genealogical evidence, interpretive claims are made and supported by reference to evidence from the analysis. The reader of a genealogy should have a clear picture of what the author claims happened with respect to power in the development of the discourse being analyzed.

STRUCTURAL ANALYSIS

Foucault advised (Dreyfus and Rabinow, 1983, appendix) that in order to conduct a discourse analysis, the following general issues within the structure of a discourse must be addressed:

1. the "system of differentiations" or privileged access to the discourse,
2. the "types of objectives" of one group over another,
3. the "means of bringing power relations into being" that reveals surveillance systems, threats, and dismissals,
4. "forms of institutionalization" such as bureaucratic structures, and
5. "degree of rationalization" required to support power arrangements.

Foucault did not conceptualize a discourse as a separate unified whole (Mish'alani, 1988). A discourse does have, however, inherent nonrandom contradictions. The contradictions are ordered by certain rules, stated or unstated. There is no necessary unity to the set of theoretical concepts that concern a discourse. There is no static repertoire of concepts in a discourse. There is no single style of statement. There is no unalterable structure to the four components of a discourse, the subjects, the objects, the styles of statements, and the theoretical strategies. What is important to know about structure of a discourse is the *regularity* or the *rules* that govern the array of diversity within these four components of a discourse (Mish'alani, 1988).

The objects of a discourse are the entities considered to be external to the discourse that are viewed as the targets for knowledge generation and intervention in a foundational manner. The objects of a discourse are described and thus constructed by the processes of the discourse, forming its subjects.

The subjects of a discourse are constructed by the discourse from the objects by being manipulated in systematic ways. This is to say that objects are external targets and subjects are internal concepts, sometimes referred to in research terminology as variables. Subjects are constructed from objects by the social and discursive processes of the discourse focused on what is assumed to be an objectively existing entity.

The styles of statements in a discourse are the forms that meaningful statements can take. The theoretical strategies are the forms that the processes of the discourse are allowed to take. The style of statements and theoretical strategies are determined by the genealological history of the discourse, the assumptions of the discourse, and by the resulting discursive practices of the discourse.

The regularities that govern the multiplicity and diversity of the four components can also be described in another way. The multiplicity and diversity of these components can be described by the implicit order that governs the rules for the appearance, disappearance, replacement, and coexistence of each of the four components in a discourse (Mish'alani, 1988, p. 13).

For example, consider the rules for the formation (appearance) of subjects in a discourse from its objects. There are three dimensions along which objects become subjects in a discourse: (1) surfaces of emergence, (2) authorities of delimitation, and (3) grids of specification. The rules for the construction of subjects are explicated by describing the ways these three dimensions are used. Subjects in a discourse multiply because there are rules within the discourse that describe what can count as subjects and objects, what sorts of things can seriously be said about them, who can say them, and what concepts can be used to say them (Dreyfus and Rabinow, 1983, p. 71).

A surface of emergence can be thought of as the contiguous edge of a body of discourse that has implications that allow tangential discourses to arise, as it were, on its surface (Foucault, 1975). A discourse arises in relation to other ways of thinking, not in some independent manner. For example, the discourse of medicine arose on the surfaces of emergence called natural science and philosophy. The styles of statements in medicine follow the rules of biology. Theoretical strategies in medicine are based on foundational empirical analytic science and require strict research protocols.

An authority of delimitation is another discourse that sets limits on the identification of subjects for the discourse in question. An authority of delimitation for the discipline of nursing is medicine, because medicine is the authority that identifies cases for the discourse of nursing to consider.

A grid of specification is a systematic discursive ordering of concepts constructed within the discourse. An example of a grid of specification is a taxonomy for subjects in a discourse. In psychiatry, for example, one of the grids of specification is the DSM-IV. In this example, the objects of the discourse are the presumed physical and behavioral states described by the diagnoses. The subjects of the discourse are the psychiatric diagnoses. It is assumed that the states (the objects) described by the diagnoses of the discourse (the subjects) actually exist in some objective way in an uninterpreted foundational reality.

Within this grid of specification the different diagnoses are divided from one another by definitions classified, interrelated, and placed in a taxonomy. The diagnoses are then used in clinical practice on preexisting surfaces or physical spaces (in this case, individual human bodies or groups of bodies such as families), which also have been described by the discursive practices of the discourse in certain regularized and normalized ways that help determine the practices and outcomes. Desirable and undesirable outcomes are specified, treatments are proposed, tested, and evaluated with respect to the descriptions acceptable to the discipline, and the discourse expands.

Bodies are the surfaces of emergence in this example, and they constitute the context within which people's individual differences, deviations, and complaints are noted by the discursive practices of the discipline. Examples of these individual differences in psychiatry include family dynamics and the community context. Both grids of specification and surfaces of emergence are coordinated by psychiatry in collaboration with the authorities for the delimitation and identification of cases such as courts, medicine, nursing, religious authorities, employers, families, and school officials. Authorities of delimitation are sometimes termed *referral sources.*

In the accepted relations among the rules for the appearance of subjects, psychiatry manipulates its constructed subjects using scientific discourse. Scientific work provides the evidence for the manipulation of the diagnoses, forming them, deforming, preserving, deriving, altering, replacing, and effacing them.

In this one arena of rules (the appearance, construction, or formation of subjects), we can see the interconnectedness of discourse to institutional structures (clinics and hospitals), nondiscursive practices (rituals and assumptions), and power relations (professional to professional, and professional to client). The other areas of regularities in the formation of subjects besides the rules for the formation or appearance of subjects are the rules for the formation of styles of statements and the rules for the formation of theoretical strategies.

Knowledge and power are so closely interrelated that the field of operation of a discourse is coextensive with a field of power. Since discourse is so closely linked to other social practices, it is easy to see why there can be so many contradictions and tensions between them within a single discourse.

In psychiatry, for example, there is incommensurability between the discourses of medicine and psychology with respect to the subjects of the discourse of psychiatry—the diagnoses. Competition among subdiscourses based on different kinds of scientific evidence for the cause of bipolar disorder, for example, gets played out within the intradisciplinary discourse and its system of power/knowledge. These competing subdiscourses are identified from a power perspective in a discourse analysis, and their relative strengths and weaknesses are discussed.

The interrelatedness of one discourse to other discourses, institutions, and practices makes it impossible to totally restrict consideration to one discourse or another. A discourse analyst could not analyze a discourse in nursing without referring to the discourse of medicine because the power relations between the two disciplines are so interrelated. Furthermore, it is impossible to retreat to a compromise position outside of the discourses under discussion in order to determine some essence to which to appeal in order to justify conclusions concerning the field of power relations.

The discursive practices of a discourse produce the subjects from the objects. The subjects of the discourse arise within the "space" or on the "surface of emergence" that was appropriated, named, and made visible by the original discursive practices. The discourse combines various practices in a unified way in a certain space, both constituting and being constituted by these practices. This process can also be viewed as the discipline "carving out a turf" for itself among other disciplines, physical spaces, power relations, theoretical orientations, talk, action, and social processes.

Rawlinson (1987) provides a compact summary of the Foucaultian approach to structural discourse analysis. According to Rawlinson, a functioning discourse may be conceptualized as the horizon of thought for a participant in that discourse (p. 375). The identifying features of this horizon are the concepts, rules, and authorities that determine the discourse. According to Rawlinson (1987, p. 377), the structural part of a discourse analysis is elaborated on three axes. First is the axis of knowledge which includes analysis of the system of concepts and rules for the formation of statements. The axis also includes the rules for determining true and false, often called the "method" of the discourse, which is acknowledged to have the power to produce truth in the discourse. This is a structural analysis that includes the rules of evidence and rules concerning what can be addressed and what cannot be addressed. Rawlinson calls this the closed system of truth within the discourse.

Second is the axis of authority. This axis includes analysis of the rules for the determination of who has the right to speak in the discourse; systems for the preservation, transmission, and general dissemination of the discourse; rules for establishing the relative authority of the discourse vis-à-vis other discourses; and systems of education and association for the reproduction and advancement of members of the discourse. The discourse analyst describes how the right to pronounce truth is preserved, exercised, and reproduced. The discourse establishes these things internally. This is the system of power/knowledge.

The third axis is the axis of value or justification. The important structures in this axis are the systems of regulation, organization, normalization, and punishment, and the technologies of power. The discourse analyst describes how the deployment of the disciplinary or normalizing strategies on the bodies of human beings is justified within the discourse. Not only does the discourse constitute something (the subjects of the discourse) by describing the subjects from the objects in the way it has set for itself, but also the discourse produces something when viewed from a power perspective. The discourse generalizes its subjects, producing an ideal, a standard, the regular, the normal, through its work. Then the discourse functions in a policing role to maintain the range of normal that it has described, by power and control, utilizing appropriately trained social agents who have been educated to think of themselves as participating in the advancement of civilization and the betterment of humankind. Rawlinson calls this the closed system of value, which is necessarily political.

To return to the example of psychiatry, the discourse defines the normal range of psychological behavior and determines the dividing line between normal and abnormal. The policing, normalizing social function of psychiatry arises from the power to classify behavior as normal or abnormal and is upheld by social conventions that assign consequences to the action of diagnosis. Such consequences, in the case of psychiatry, may include involuntary medication and/or incarceration. Rawlinson's explication provides for the formulation of questions based on what is important in the analysis of each of these axes.

The structural part of the discourse analysis therefore answers the following questions:

On the axis of knowledge: What are the objects and subjects of the discourse? What processes differentiate the subjects and objects of the discourse? What is it that guides this discourse? What regularities can be discerned? What processes produce the physical space, the meaning, and the assumed truths of this discourse? What does the discourse do to the resulting subjects? What grids of specification are there? In the rules for the formation of subjects from objects, what and where do individual differences, deviations, and complaints emerge? How is it specified that these subjects are to be used on preexisting surfaces, constructed spaces, or bodies? What authorities of delimitation exist? What order governs the appearance, disappearance, replacement, and coexistence of the subjects, objects, concepts, styles of statements, and theoretical strategies of the discourse? What are the rules of evidence in the discourse? What order governs the multiplicity and diversity of the subjects, objects, concepts, styles of statements, and theoretical strategies of the discourse?

On the axis of authority: The analysis of the axis of authority asks how the discourse preserves its socially constructed right to pronounce truth in some realm of human experience and how the discourse is transmitted within its social position. What are the rules for who is allowed to speak and who is not? How is the discourse preserved, transmitted, and disseminated? What systems are allowed for education, association, and advancement of members of the discourse? How is the right to pronounce truth preserved? What speaking positions are available to people within this discourse? What speaking positions are not allowed?

On the axis of value or justification: The analysis of the axis of value or justification asks how the discourse justifies the technologies of power that it constructs for its purposes and how the discourse justifies suppressing other discourses that challenge its dominance in pronouncing truth. How are the technologies of power/knowledge justified by the discourse? What justification is provided for the punishment of participants? How is the suppression of competing discourses justified? What is the justification provided by the discourse for its position as a pronouncer of truth?

The answers to these questions produce the structural analysis. The answers describe the present functioning of the discourse with respect to its genealogy and the resulting rules, implicit and explicit, of its practice and continued existence. Other questions can be asked and answered, according to the situation of the discourse.

POWER ANALYSIS OR ANALYTIC

Given the first two portions, the genealogy and the structural discourse analysis, the relations of power supported by the discourse are analyzed for the potential to perpetuate or extend situations of domination for individuals and/or groups. Alternative potential speaking positions within the discourse are identified as possible ways of constructing subjectivities that may give rise to practices of resistance to the domination effects of the discourse. These potential speaking positions provide ways of speaking and acting that do not support the dominant meaning-making activity.

The process of conducting a power analysis (also called power analytic) involves careful reading of the discourse with a view to discerning discursive patterns of meaning, contradictions, and inconsistencies (Weedon, 1987) that illuminate power relations. The analysis identifies language processes and social practices that people use to constitute their subjective existences and to construct their understanding of social life. These processes either reproduce or challenge the distribution of power as it currently exists (p. 467).

A power analytic accounts for the social production of identities and institutional orders that frequently are assumed to be natural; they aim to free individuals from essentialist identities that constrain behavior; they strive to unearth submerged alternative languages to describe experiences and open up new possibilities for social identification and behavior. (Seidman, 1992, p. 70)

Influenced by postmodernism, a power analytic shows how social power is constructed, circulated, and played out (Seidel, 1993, p. 175).

Foucault did not include claims regarding the preferability of some situations of domination or resistance over others. In other versions of discourse analysis, however, preferability of speaking positions and practices may be identified. Specific practices of resistance may be openly advocated. The feminist perspective on discourse analysis is one that acknowledges the possibility and desirability of the creation of new options, new speaking positions, which, in turn, form new subjectivities, or new ideologies with new limits and new possibilities (McIntosh, 1988). Other authors argue that a discourse analyst may acknowledge new options and speaking positions without advocating a preference for one over another (Traynor, 1997).

Naming and describing resistance can, however, initiate the discourse's own process of co-optation and control based on the goal of emancipation. During such examination as takes place in a power analysis, feminist process variables assume critical importance in the identification of positions of power and resistance in the power analytic of a particular instance of domination. From a feminist perspective, a power analytic includes a focus on oppression, how powerless groups are oppressed within power relations, the possibilities of resistance, and how marginalized voices can attempt to challenge dominant discourses. Using an antifoundational perspective, discourse analysis assumes that people can be deceived about what is going on, without having to assume that it is possible or even desirable to know what is "really" going on. The discourse can be analyzed for the existence of respect for diversity of perspectives and the inclusion of the voices of the people addressed by the discourse. Whose voice is privileged in this discourse?

A power analytic may involve identification of several discourses available to people in a given situation at a given time (Gavey, 1989). An analysis of this type will show how the discourse provides alternative speaking positions (Gavey, 1989) that function either to reproduce or challenge existing power relations. Some of these alternative speaking positions may be termed *marginalized discourses*. Marginalized discourses are nondominant discourses that may include (or be influenced by) discourses or practices of resistance. When marginal discourses come under scrutiny by more powerful discourses, the possibility exists that they may be co-opted into the dominant discourse. Sometimes marginalized discourses are co-opted without much alteration, in which case they may be said to have been *incorporated*. On the other hand, the marginalized discourse may undergo extensive alterations by being co-opted, which renders it completely sterile as an alternative subject position available to people.

A power analytic acknowledges the ability of individuals to recognize power relations and the ways in which their options are limited by their own beliefs. In addition, the capacity of people for activities of resistance and the possibility of co-optation are also acknowledged. Systematic limitations can be brought to light whether or not they are identified as dominant or marginal. The political and power effects of the discourse analysis itself cannot be ignored.

In the power analysis part of a discourse analysis, the following questions are asked: In whose interests are the continuation of this discourse? Whose autonomy and responsibility are enhanced by this discourse? Whose autonomy and responsibility are reduced? What dominations are established, perpetuated, or eliminated? What subdiscourses of resistance are present within the discourse? What mechanisms are in place for systematic co-optation of resistance discourses? Whose voice is being heard? Whose voice is being left out? Do people feel constraints against speaking? Are all voices equally informed? What power relations exist between this discourse and others?

The answers to these questions form the power analysis of the discourse analysis. Placement of the discourse within the social web of power in a situated context for concerned individuals can produce insights and can give people new ways to think and talk about the discourses in which they function.

THE EVALUATION OF RIGOR
AND SCHOLARSHIP

Methodological differences among discourse analyses exist. Consider the small child who, when told that she was not printing proper A's, said, "Well, that's how I make A's!" and received the answer that "This would be fine if you were the only person who reads what you write." Variations in personal style can still be understandable to others, but adherence to the current standards of social meaning and logic are required for any analysis to hold up to scrutiny by others. You cannot print A's and expect everyone to read P's. A discourse analyst would not read in a discourse over and over again that male immigrants were systematically excluded from taking part in the discourse and then in the end make the claim that "male immigrants constituted the major portion of the practitioners." Being complete, honest, consistent, and systematic and using the currently accepted procedure for drawing inferences, making claims, and supporting interpretations using appropriate data are as important in a discourse analysis as they are in any well argued position. No assumption is made that the standards of western Greek-based logic and argumentation are universally applicable to all cultures and times, but the general audience for works of this nature construct meaning on this basis. For a further discussion of the crises of authority and representation, see Denzin (1997).

The question may then be asked, "What's the difference between this method of analysis and a historical investigation or a conceptual study or a piece of investigative reporting or a popular novel?" There are overlaps, to be sure, but the major answer is the positive focus on power and the lack of focus on theory, events, and the deeds of great people. An historical account answers the question, "What happened?" while a discourse analysis answers, "What power relations are involved in the history and present functioning of this discourse?"

A history of piano making, for example, would detail the construction of the first piano, its predecessors and successors, the lives of great piano makers, the refinements and evolution of piano making, and so on. A discourse analysis of piano making would focus on the gaze instead of the objects being illuminated by the gaze. A discourse of piano making would detail the conditions of possibility for piano making such as the availability of certain kinds of wood, strings, and so on. It would discuss the influence of audience size and the audibility of previous stringed instruments compared to a piano. It would discuss the composition of the group of people who made the first pianos and would ask the following questions: How is it that these people made pianos and other people did not? In whose interests were the making of pianos? Who did and did not benefit from piano making? How was the knowledge of piano making passed along? What justified the expense of making a piano compared to making a zither or a harp?

LIMITATIONS

The limitations of discourse analysis arise from the methodology on which it is based. Since no claim is made for the absolute truth of the claims made in a discourse analysis, one of the limitations is that other, competing claims are possible regarding the same discourse. This seems like a serious limitation until one considers that the same limitation applies to other methods of inquiry as well. Any scientific study of, for example, the genetic cause of schizophrenia may be followed by an equally well performed study that refutes the evidence and provides compelling evidence for a viral cause of schizophrenia. A sociological analysis of the breast feeding of infants among rural Canadian women may be contradicted by another team of researchers in the same part of the country. An article on cold fusion may be refuted by another article. A historical novel is critiqued by another historical novel. The point is that there is a progression of publications and analyses and critiques that is ongoing among members of academic disciplines according to social rules. In 50 years, there will probably be a discourse analysis of the discourse of discourse analysis that describes the implicit and explicit regularities that govern the rules for conducting a discourse analysis.

GENERALIZABILITY

The results of a discourse analysis are not generalizable to other situations, other discourses, or other people. If an analyst reads a compelling discourse analysis of the discourse of computer software writers and wonders if the same things can be said regarding computer hardware designers, then that person would have to do the discourse analysis (or assign the project to a graduate student) to find out.

CONSEQUENCES, EFFECTS, AND DURABILITY

The discourse analyst always hopes that the work will raise the consciousness of the readers and inform the work of people within the discourse in order to reduce oppression and provide alternate speaking positions. It is possible that the analysis itself will have unintended consequences and/or will result in the co-optation of resistance discourses and/or not reach the people who would understand and benefit from the work.

The concept of audience is crucial to the discourse analyst, as it should be to other researchers. Where is the emancipatory potential of a discourse analysis if no one hears about it? Publication of discourse analyses usually reaches other members of the discourse in which the analyst participates and may miss the people in the discourse that was analyzed. When a discourse analyst asks, "Whose interests are being served by the operation of this discourse?" shouldn't the analyst also ask, "Whose interests would be served by reading this discourse analysis?" Social action is informed by discourse and should be informed by discourse analyses as well. To that end, a discourse analyst should make more of an effort at dissemination of findings than members of other research traditions.

Feminist researchers often take drafts or presentations back to the research subjects or informants before publication. This is done to ask the participants whether or not the researcher, made valid interpretations. Be prepared for conflicting feedback, and then reflect the conflict in the final version. Remember, even the Supreme Court allows "minority opinions." Group research often results in different interpretations that can be very enlightening to readers (see Cheek & Gibson, 1996).

Publication should include professional literature but should also include some method of dissemination that reaches people that would benefit from the analysis. This may necessitate revision into a style that would be more easily understood by readers. An academic paper entitled "A Discourse Analysis of Personal Athletic Trainers" is fine for the imaginary *Journal of Sports Medicine*, but an article called "Why Do Personal Athletic Trainers Talk the Way They Do?" would be more appropriate for *Woman's Day* magazine.

The durability and sustainability of the results of a discourse analysis are affected by several considerations. A discourse analysis does not purport to reveal absolute truth. Situations change, discourses change, power relations shift, and other discourse analyses are published. Another discourse analysis of the same discourse may be indicated. It would be sad to think that the same analysis would apply to the discourse of, Asian American kindergarten teachers in 20 years as it does today. If it did, it might indicate that the same dominant and resistance discourses are operating without insight, concepts are not being problematized, issues are not being discussed, and new voices are not being heard. Discourse analyses are written in order to become rewritten.

REFERENCES

Cheek, J., & Gibson, T. (1996). The discursive construction of the role of the nurse in medication administration: An exploration of the literature. *Nursing Inquiry*, 3(3), 83–90.

Denzin, N. K. (1997). *Interpretive ethnography: Ethnographic practices of the* 21st century. Thousand Oaks, CA: Sage.

Denzin, N. K., & Lincoln, Y. S. (2000). *Handbook of Qualitative Research* (2nd ed.). Thousand Oaks, CA: Sage.

Dreyfus, H. (1987). Foucault's critique of psychiatric medicine. *Journal of Medicine and Philosophy*, 12(4), 311–333.

Dreyfus, H., & Rabinow, P. (1983). *Michel Foucault, beyond structuralism and hermeneutics.* Chicago: University of Chicago Press.

Fields: An investigation into archaeological and genealogical science studies. Dordrecht, The Netherlands: Kluwer Academic Publishers.

Foss, S. K., & Gill, A. (1987). Michel Foucault's theory of rhetoric as epistemic. *Western Journal of Speech Communication, 51,* 384–401.

Foucault, M. (1975). *The birth of the clinic.* Translated by A. M. Sheridan-Smith. New York: Vintage/Random House.

Foucault, M. (1977). *Knowledge, counter-memory, and practice: Selected essays and interviews* (D. F. Bouchard, Ed.). Ithaca, NY: Cornell Press.

Foucault, M. (1979). *Discipline and punish: The birth of the prison,* (A. Sheridan, Trans.). New York: Vintage/Random House.

Gavey, N. (1989). Feminist poststructuralism and discourse analysis. *Psychology of Women Quarterly, 13,* 459–475.

Kusch, M. (1991). *Foucault's Strata and Fields: An investigation into archaeological and genealogical science studies.* Dordrecht, The Netherlands: Kluwer Academic Publishers.

McIntosh, P. (1988). *White privilege and male privilege: A personal account of coming to see correspondences through work in women's studies, Working Paper No. 189.* Wellesley, MA: Wellesley College.

Mish'alani, J. K. (1988). Michel Foucault and philosophy: An overview. Unpublished paper. University of Washington at Seattle.

Rawlinson, M. (1987). Foucault's strategy: Knowledge, power, and the specificity of truth. *Journal of Medicine and Philosophy, 12*(4), 372–395.

Seidel, G. (1993). The competing discourses of HIV/AIDS in sub-Saharan Africa: Discourses of rights and empowerment vs. discourses of control and exclusion. *Social Sciences and Medicine, 36*(3), 175–194.

Seidman, S. (1992). Postmodern social theory as narrative with a moral intent. In S. Seidman & D. Wagner (Eds.), *Postmodernism and social theory.* Cambridge, MA: Blackwell.

Traynor, M. (1997). Postmodern research: No grounding or privilege, just free-floating trouble making. *Nursing Inquiry, 4*(2), 99–107.

Weedon, C. (1987). *Feminist practice and poststructuralist theory.* Oxford: Blackwell.

CHAPTER 4

A DISCOURSE ANALYSIS OF NURSING DIAGNOSIS

INTRODUCTION

This chapter presents an example of a discourse analysis from the discipline of nursing. This discourse analysis of "nursing diagnosis" in nursing literature and practice in the United States follows the method described in chapter 3. The analysis contains an introduction, a genealogy, a structural analysis, and a power analysis.

The controversial idea of nurses assigning a "nursing diagnosis" to a patient that is different from a medical diagnosis first appeared in the U.S. nursing literature in the 1950s and became increasingly prevalent up to the early 1990s. Since the failure of national health care reform in the United States and the rise of managed care, the concept and use of nursing diagnosis has become less prevalent. Nursing diagnosis appeared in the American Nursing Association's (ANA) Standards of Practice document, it appeared in the Joint Commission accreditation requirements for hospitals in the United States, and then it disappeared again. In addition, the North American Nursing Diagnosis Association (NANDA) has held national conferences, and a journal called *Nursing Diagnosis* is available for research in nursing diagnosis and related topics.

Within any discipline, the empirical truth claims of prominent discourses are subjected to analysis more often than the more abstract dimensions. Ethical, ideological, and power-related meta-issues commonly receive less attention in intradisciplinary literature. The discourse of nursing diagnosis has received very little critique and no systematic analysis.

The methodology is antifoundational in the sense that discourse analysis is consistent with a position opposed to the foundational assumptions of the empirical analytic tradition of scientific inquiry. The methodology can be said to be postmodern because it rejects the assumption of a value-neutral foundation of empirical facts for the social sciences. This discourse analysis is feminist because it asks whether the discourse demonstrates systematic effects with respect to socially defined categories such as race, class, and gender.

The analysis will be presented in three sections: a genealogy, a structural discourse analysis, and a power analytic. These three sections are closely related and overlapping but are presented separately for conceptual clarity.

GENEALOGY

A genealogy examines the major influences on the development of a discourse. The text for this genealogy consisted of all published articles, books, accounts, and comments on nursing diagnosis up to the first national conference in 1973. The genealogy of nursing diagnosis revealed several influential bodies of knowledge. The models or discourses on which the discourse of nursing diagnosis was based were identified as medicine, foundational science, and professionalism.

The definition of *profession* is

> an occupation which has assumed a dominant position in a division of labor, so that it gains control over the determination of the substance of its own work . . . it claims to be the most reliable authority on the nature of the reality it deals with . . . [it] changes the definition and shape of the problems as experienced by the layman. The layman's problem is re-created as it is managed—a new social reality is created by . . . the autonomous position of the profession in society." (Friedson, 1970, p. xvii)

The origin and development of the concept of *diagnosis* in the English language with respect to medicine is a key consideration in a genealogy of nursing diagnosis. Definitions and redefinitions always constitute a move related to social power (Allen, 1986). The implications of the choice of the word *diagnosis* for the discourse of nursing diagnosis are pervasive. The subdiscourses and models implied by the choice of this word inform the structure and functioning of the discourse of nursing diagnosis. Thus, it is instructive to review the development of the word *diagnosis* in medicine.

Two conceptual facets of the idea of diagnosis in the practice of medicine can also be identified within the discourse of nursing diagnosis. Describing these facets underscores the imitation of medical diagnosis by nursing diagnosis. In dealing with the resulting tension, the discourse of nursing diagnosis will be shown to perpetuate the same power inequities at the expense of the practice of nursing itself.

The *Oxford English Dictionary* (1989) defines the word *diagnosis* as follows:

> Greek, noun, meaning "of action" from the Greek word "to distinguish, or discern" which comes from two other Greek words, one meaning "thoroughly asunder" and the other meaning "to learn to know or perceive." 1. In medicine it is the determination of the nature

of a diseased condition; identification of a disease by careful investigation of its symptoms and history. 2. The opinion resulting from the investigation.

Diagnoses are not immutable entities in an absolutely knowable reality, but dynamic social and historical constructions (Bynum & Nutton, 1981).

It is important to note in this definition that to diagnose is not to decide between health and nonhealth states but involves the discerning of the name of a nonhealthy state. The purpose of the action of diagnosis is the discerning of what kind of nonhealth a person is experiencing, instead of whether the person is healthy or not healthy. The action of diagnosis has, therefore, the socially influential power of naming.

In ancient Greece, two schools of thought with respect to diagnosis and treatment existed. In one, discerning the prognosis of a patient was more important than naming the phenomenon. Naming and classifying diseases were considered philosophical enterprises, not clinical tasks. These physicians prescribed treatments according to symptoms and criticized others for "multiplying types and assigning essential importance to accidental details" (Galdston, 1981, p. 55).

The other school of thought concentrated on the classification of specifically named diseases according to minute individual variations of signs and symptoms, each variation being productive of another species of disease. These physicians then prescribed treatments according to named and classified disease entities, accusing the first group of physicians of being more concerned with individual clinical circumstances than advancing general knowledge.

These two orientations to diagnosis have continued to influence various factions in medical research to this day (Galdston, 1981). Galdston emphasized the difference between the perspectives as follows:

> To diagnose a disease as a distinct entity is a more primitive function. It requires but a moderate mental discipline. It can frequently be accomplished by using inanimate instruments. It offers only a narrow and none too stable foundation for effective therapy. . . . Diagnosis practiced as the definition of a clinical problem affecting a given individual, to be solved therapeutically, is by far the superior and more difficult function. (p. 56)

These two different approaches to diagnosis, which have informed medicine for over 2,000 years, also have had a profound effect on the discipline of nursing in general and the discourse of nursing diagnosis in particular. The tension between these two approaches to medical diagnosis has been re-created in the discourse of nursing diagnosis by the choice of the word *diagnosis* without acknowledging the problematic issues associated with the notion in medicine.

One important unintended consequence of this re-creation is that the assumptions have continued to inform the discourse of nursing diagnosis in the same way as they inform the discourse of medical diagnosis. That is to say that the tension between the two approaches to diagnosis obscures the operation of the following assumptions that underlie both the medical and nursing concept of diagnosis: (1) the entity diagnosed has an objective existence apart from our understanding of it, and (2) the name given to the entity somehow captures the essence of that entity as it exists within people in an objective world. Noting the tension between the opposing goals of adding to general knowledge (science) and treating individual clinical circumstances (practice) will help to illuminate the power relations between academic and practicing nurses and between nursing and health care systems.

Now consider the social context of the discipline of nursing in the 1950s, the time when the concept of nursing diagnosis was being addressed in the United States. This is important because it illuminates the range of options available as models for the goals of the discipline. At this time, there were very few nurses with advanced degrees, and these degrees were predominantly in other disciplines such as education or sociology. Medicine was the preeminent model of a profession in U.S. culture. The empirical analytic tradition was the only model of science generally available, marginalized discourses such as critical theory and phenomenology notwithstanding.

In post-World War II America, nurses returning from military service had increased skills in treating medical diagnoses in cooperation with physicians. Returning to peacetime practice, nurses faced renewed domination from physicians and social pressure to return to traditionally defined female roles with reduced status in order to make room for returning male soldiers into the workforce.

Consequently, nurses felt increased pressure to redefine their unique status and value. This goal had been articulated in various forms since 1900 (Turkoski, 1992), but after World War II the drive intensified and many nurses went back to school. The discourses of medicine and science constituted the desirable discourses available to nursing (and anyone else) that could be used to describe value, power, and status in the modern post-war social world of the 1950s. Using these discourses as models and using professional status as a goal, nursing diagnosis was constructed.

McManus (1951) and Fry (1953) advocated the discipline-specific term *nursing diagnosis* in nursing literature and suggested adoption of care plans to guide nursing practice, based on a model of human needs from psychology. In 1956, Hornung argued that occupational health nurses are often called upon to make medical diagnoses, which she called "nursing diagnoses," when there is no physician in attendance to do so (1956, p. 29).

There were very few nursing diagnosis articles published in the 1960s, and differing definitions were used (see summary in Edel, 1982). During the 1960s, the terms *problem* and *need* were more prevalent than the term *diagnosis*, but all three terms referred to an "independent" function of nursing, the use of which, it was felt, would cause "vague descriptions of the patient's condition [to] disappear from our vocabulary" (Hornung, 1956, p. 30).

During the late 1950s and early 1960s, the term *science* was applied to nursing, which had an important influence on the discourse of nursing diagnosis. An early instance of the term *nursing science* in nursing literature is found in the earliest work of Martha Rogers, published in 1963. She argued that nursing constituted a unique body of knowledge and that the application of this body of knowledge constituted the practice of nursing. Abdellah (1969) also called nursing a science and argued that the ability to make diagnoses is fundamental to the development of any science. Jacox (1974) described the classification of concepts as one of the first steps in theory development in any science.

McFarland and McFarlane (1993) emphasized the importance of this decade in the development of the discourse of nursing diagnosis, noting that an article published by a doctor in the *Journal of the American Medical Association* in 1967 defined diagnosis in general terms not specific to medicine. This article (King, 1967) defines criteria or components that must be present to make a diagnosis:

1. There must be a preexisting series of categories or classes that provide a reference for the diagnosis.
2. There must be a particular entity that is to be diagnosed.
3. There must be a deliberate judgment that the assessed phenomenon or response belongs in the particular category or class.

McFarland and McFarlane (1993) implied that this article was the impetus for the first NANDA conference. Douglas and Murphy (1990) noted that another article with respect to the concept of scientific classification by *Sokal in Science* in 1974 was also an early influence on efforts towards the classification of nursing diagnoses (p. 17).

With hindsight, Gebbie (in foreword to Carlson, Craft, & McGuire, 1982), co-chair of the first national conference on nursing diagnosis, identified some other influences on the historical development of the discourse:

No group of health care providers could expect increased public support, increased professional respect, or increased monetary reward unless that group was known to have a direct impact on the health of the nation's citizens and was able to demonstrate clear quality control on the care provided. . . . A concise universal language of nursing diagnoses could provide a frame for the needed demonstration. (p. vii)

The major discourse, the daily practice language of nursing, has been and remains medical (Street, 1992). The concept of nursing diagnosis had the appeal of combining the socially desirable and powerful discourses of medicine, science, and professionalism that were major models of social authority, power, and value in the 1950s and 1960s and remain so today.

Historically, nursing has vacillated between highlighting differences and highlighting similarities between itself and medicine, according to the ideological purpose served by each position in a specific historical context. The concept of nursing diagnosis had the advantage of being able to emphasize both the similarities and the differences at the same time. As stated by Edel, "medical and nursing diagnoses differ in as much as medicine and nursing differ and are similar in as much as medicine and nursing are similar" (1982, p. 7).

The concept of nursing diagnosis was subsequently incorporated into a component of the nursing process, which was incorrectly perceived at the time to be a variant of the foundational empirical analytic scientific method (Douglas & Murphy, 1990; Hiraki, 1992). The nursing process was first advocated in nursing literature by Hall (1955). The four-step nursing process consisted of assessment, planning, implementation, and evaluation of nursing care (Yura & Walsh, 1973). Nursing diagnosis was added in the 1970s and usually was placed at the end of the assessment phase or the beginning of the planning phase (Douglas & Murphy, 1990; Stelzer & Becker, 1982). A five-step nursing process added the step of nursing diagnosis between the assessment and planning phases. Early proponents of this five-step process were Roy (1975), Aspinal (1976), and Mundinger and Jauron (1975).

Nursing diagnosis and nursing process were viewed as the means to mediate between theory and practice. Nursing used the discourse of nursing process to standardize the concept of nursing care, hoping that it would help to earn professional status (Gebbie & Lavin, 1975, p. 23; Hiraki, 1992, p. 130). McFarland and McFarlane (1993) argued that nursing diagnosis was the critical link in the nursing process because "the symptoms of conditions diagnosed can be alleviated or modified by nursing actions" (p. 11). Nursing diagnosis, however, also has been called the weakest component of the nursing process (Andersen & Briggs, 1988; Aspinal, 1976).

Many purposes have been cited for the original development of the discourse of nursing diagnosis. The array of purposes clearly shows the tension between the two views of the diagnostic process, the provision of general knowledge and guidance in individual practice situations. Two of the purposes for developing the language of nursing diagnosis have been identified as the provision of a precise language for practice (Levine, 1989) and a language for theory development (Edel, 1982).

In the proceedings of the third and fourth NANDA conferences, Kim and Moritz (1982) offered the following assessment of the original impetus for nursing diagnosis:

> The conferences . . . proceed on the assumption that nurses diagnose as part of their professional activity and that nurses are seeking guidance in clearly and accurately articulating the nursing diagnoses they make and in further understanding the theoretical framework on which these diagnoses are based. (p. xviii)

This claim that the development of the discourse of nursing diagnosis was initiated and influenced by "nurses seeking guidance" was questioned in later conferences and will be discussed later with respect to the domination of academics over practitioners.

Another original purpose for the development of nursing diagnosis was identified by Gebbie and Lavin (1975) at the first conference. The increasing influence of hospital computers was thought to demand a standardized language from nurses (Saba, 1989). Levine argued further that the process of creating this standardized nursing language was meant to be accomplished through clinicians sharing real-life clinical experiences (1989, p. 5).

Efficiency, standardization, and accountability are also cited as influences on the development of the discourse of nursing diagnosis (Edel, 1982, p. 8). Nursing diagnosis was seen as the approach that could provide the "frame of reference from which nurses could determine (1) what to do and (2) what to expect" in a clinical practice situation (Edel, 1982, p. 9).

Nursing diagnoses were also intended to define nursing's unique boundaries with respect to medical diagnoses (Douglas & Murphy, 1990; Pridham & Schutz, 1985). Harrington (1988), for example, argued that nursing diagnosis was the defining characteristic of nursing practice. This argument was based on the ANA's 1980 social policy statement, which defined nursing as the diagnosis and treatment of human responses. "The issue of validity of nursing diagnoses holds the key to verifying nursing practice and therefore to fulfilling the profession's social responsibility to render effective, cost-effective care" (Derdiarian, 1988, p. 140). On the basis of this judgment, NANDA meant the standardization of nursing language to be the first step toward having insurance companies pay nurses directly for their care (Carpenito, 1989; Edel, 1982; Gebbie & Lavin, 1975, p. 23; Gordon, 1982a, p. 284; Webb, 1992).

In order to demonstrate the influence of social discourses as models of power for the development of nursing diagnosis, consider the following early definitions of nursing diagnosis, which were prior to the first NANDA conference:

1. "Nursing diagnosis is the identification of the nursing problem and the recognition of its interrelated aspects" (McManus, 1951, p. 54).
2. "The determination of the nature and extent of nursing problems presented by the individual patients or families receiving nursing care" (Abdellah, 1957, p. 4).
3. "A careful investigation of the facts to determine the nature of a nursing problem" (Chambers, 1962, p. 102). A problem was defined as a specific patient need, so the diagnostic process produced a linguistic statement of need for the patient.
4. "A conclusion based on scientific determination of an individual's nursing needs, resulting from critical analysis of his behavior, the nature of his illness, and numerous other factors which affect his condition. This conclusion should then serve as a guide for nursing care" (Komorita, 1963, p. 83).
5. "A statement of a conclusion resulting from a recognition of a pattern derived from a nursing investigation of the patient" (Durand & Prince, 1966, p. 51).
6. "Nursing diagnosis is determination of the nature and extent of nursing problems presented by individual patients or families receiving nursing care" (Abdellah, 1969, p. 391).

These definitions variously present the phenomena of concern to nursing as problems, needs, and/or patterns. The result of the diagnostic process is called a conclusion, a judgment, or a nursing diagnosis. In the time since these definitions were generated, the description of the phenomena of concern to nursing still has not been clarified, despite the ANA's use of the term *human responses* in 1980. Tension between the goals of general knowledge provision and clinical practice are clearly represented in the words used to describe what it is that concerns nurses.

From a genealogical perspective, the discourse of nursing diagnosis arose in a social context utilizing both surfaces of emergence and conditions of possibility that were acknowledged and appropriated and made visible by the emerging discourse on nursing diagnosis. One surface of emergence for the discourse of nursing diagnosis was the change from an emphasis on illness care to an emphasis on health care. The emphasis on health care focuses on health as a life goal instead of focusing on a physical state consisting simply of the absence of disease (Foucault, 1985). This orientation became one sort of language that the discourse of nursing diagnosis could use to have some kind of social meaning, power, and value because health language is tangential to disease language.

Another surface of emergence used by the discourse of nursing diagnosis is required hospital accreditation documentation. In the 1950s, trained efficiency experts were analyzing the industrial work environment in order to reduce inefficiency and to increase productivity. At the same time, in a similarly motivated move, hospital accreditation procedures began to require written documentation for assessment of quality of care. A discourse of nursing diagnosis, with scientific foundations and processes, could demonstrate nursing's contribution to the quality of care. For example, "Automated record keeping" was cited in the first conference as one of the changes in health care that necessitated a specific nursing language (Gebbie & Lavin, 1975, p. 1).

Certain conditions of possibility were appropriated by the discourse of nursing diagnosis during its development period. Conditions of possibility consist of those physical, social, and discursive circumstances that make the language of the discourse possible. One condition of possibility for the discourse of nursing diagnosis was that physicians were not always physically available in the practice environment. The nurse was the person with whom the patient had the most contact, and nurses spent more time with other nurses than they did with physicians.

In the 1950s, hospitals were using recruitment advertising that attracted nurses to work with claims of reduced patient assignments and the addition of unit clerks to reduce the amount of paperwork (Powers, 1988). This is to say that nurses spent increasingly more time talking with each other about their day-to-day practice, more time in direct patient care, and less time in administrative tasks such as answering phones. This condition of possibility meant that nurses could conceptualize their practice as qualitatively different from the practice of medicine.

Another condition of possibility was the advanced education of increasing numbers of nurses in the post-World War II science and technology boom. This education produced nurses who taught nursing, created journals in which to publish, functioned in networks, and spoke academic language. The discourse of nursing diagnosis is in large part an academic project. The first conference on nursing diagnosis was held at the St. Louis University School of Nursing and Allied Health Professions. Nursing diagnosis was expected to "facilitate research and education" (Edel, 1982, p. 8).

The surfaces of emergence and the conditions of possibility create an environment conducive to the creation of a discourse specific to the social context. Available models combined with the motivation of educated nurses in post-World War II America to redefine nursing practice in the social context of power and status to produce discursive practices. An important step in this process was the discursive creation of a physical space within which to assert the right to pronounce truth.

The discourse of nursing diagnosis, in keeping with the task of any discourse, linguistically constructs the description of a physically based, socially described space of action on bodies, using discursive processes. The physical space that is created by the discourse of nursing diagnosis will be termed the *clinical encounter* even though that phrase is not used in the discourse. Before the development of the discourse of nursing diagnosis, the meeting of a nurse and patient could be said to be determined and described by discourses other than nursing. The "nurse-patient relationship," for example, was conceived of in terms of principles from social psychology and was further refined to become a therapeutic tool for nurses to use within the clinical encounter.

The discourse of nursing diagnosis represents the attempt of the discipline of nursing to construct and take control of the clinical encounter, physically and conceptually, in order to carve out a professional turf distinct from other disciplines. Within this turf, or territory, or domain, the discourse claims the right to describe what is and what should be happening. The discourse assumes that the carving out of such a territory for itself can proceed with minimal reference to other disciplines. Bypassing discussion of the overlapping domains of disciplines creates another tension within the discourse of nursing diagnosis that will become apparent in the structural analysis.

To summarize the genealogy, it is clear that the discourse of nursing diagnosis claims the right to pronounce truth in a domain of human experience in the following manner. By utilizing conditions of possibility, appropriating surfaces of emergence, identifying influential and socially desirable discourses as models, and naming a physical space, nursing diagnosis constructed specific discursive practices. These practices created a perceived need for pronouncing truth in a move of power to further long-standing professional goals. The justification of this move using the power of redefinition was phrased in terms of the scientifically verifiable language of patient benefit and fiscal and social responsibility.

By choosing the word *diagnosis*, nursing claimed social power and status from the turf of medicine without considering the problematic issues inherent in that choice. Because of the similarities to medical diagnosis, the discourse had to clearly distinguish what nurses do and do not diagnose. By choosing the word *science*, nursing claimed expertise within the clinical encounter based on discursive practices grounded in foundational science. It was assumed that these choices would bring about the long-awaited goal of independent professionalism and the accompanying social power, money, and status. The discourse of nursing diagnosis chose imitation of the most powerful social models (science and medicine) available in the 1950s and 1960s.

STRUCTURAL ANALYSIS

The structural analysis addresses the discursive processes of the discourse of nursing diagnosis. The text for the structural analysis consisted of all of the published literature concerning the NANDA conferences because the internal rules of the discourse are largely determined by the discursive practices constructed by and through the conferences.

The conclusion of the structural analysis is that the functioning of nursing diagnosis continues to be influenced by the three models identified in the genealogy: medicine, foundational science, and professionalism. The influence of these discourses, identified in the development of the discourse, continues to influence the internal structure and functioning of the discursive practices. The power implications will be discussed in the third section of the discourse analysis, the power analytic.

THE AXIS OF KNOWLEDGE

The discourse defines as its objects of concern the *human responses* (or response patterns) *to illness*, a term introduced in the later conferences. The subjects of the discourse, the variables for manipulation that are constructed by the discourse from the objects, are the nursing diagnoses.

Rasch (1987) argued that the ANA's 1980 Social Policy Statement declares the human responses and the nursing diagnoses to be the same objective entities. Rasch (1987) also argued that the true nature of what it is that nurses diagnose has yet to be elaborated. This confusion was evident at the seventh conference, for example, when Newman (1987) argued that nurses diagnose *patterns* of human responses and not *singular* human responses. Subsequently, the name of the organizing framework for Taxonomy I was changed from *unitary man* to *human response pattern* (Carroll-Johnson, 1989).

According to the discourse of nursing diagnosis, human responses (the objects of the discourse) are assumed to be universal objective entities that exist in individual human beings in a preinterpreted objective reality. Being objective entities, the objects of the discourse are amenable to description through scientific research. The diagnoses, the subjects of the discourse, are acknowledged to be scientific constructs that linguistically represent the objective entities.

The nursing diagnoses, the subjects of the discourse, are viewed as the names of the objects in the same way that psychiatric diagnoses are often thought to be the names of conditions assumed to exist in humans and described by empirical research. From a Foucaultian perspective, both the diagnoses and the human responses (the objects and the subjects) are reified entities, statistically associated with other reified entities called causes, etiologies, determining characteristics, and so on—all described using foundational science. The process of reification fixes the description of an entity as an unchanging thing that is assumed to exist apart from its description in all human beings.

Many diagnoses take the form of an *alteration* or a *deficit* of something, such as alteration in family processes or fluid volume deficit. It was suggested at the first conference that there should be diagnoses of patient strengths as well as weaknesses (Gebbie & Lavin, 1975, p. 43), but few diagnoses of this type have been developed.

The words *situation, condition,* and *human response* are often used interchangeably for the objects of the discourse in the nursing diagnosis literature and in the conference proceedings. They have been called the focus of nursing, or nursing's unique domain (Wooldridge, Brown, & Herman, 1993). Carpenito (1993, p. 96), however, reported that she came to prefer the term "situations that necessitate nursing care" instead of "nursing diagnoses."

THE RULES FOR EMERGENCE OF SUBJECTS

The rules of the discourse specify how a diagnosis is recognized as empirically valid within the clinical encounter. There are several unacknowledged conditions inherent in the rules for the recognition of potential discursive subjects (diagnoses).

At the first conference it was stated that a "major task of all nurses is to locate those diagnoses that were neglected, to test and develop them and to present them to the profession so that they might be included in future listings" (Gebbie & Lavin, 1975, pp. 57–58). Through 1982, however, the diagnoses were still obtained through the members of NANDA and the work of a group of nursing theorists within NANDA.

Diagnoses are authorized in the following manner. In 1982, it was specified that diagnoses be proposed to a review committee, which followed a specific procedure in order to come to a conclusion to accept or reject the application for consideration. The recommendation was forwarded to a Task

Force. Acceptance of the application meant preliminary acceptance for further clinical testing, which was to be completed by nurse researchers in collaboration with clinicians.

Fawcett (1986) also encouraged each nurse interested in nursing diagnosis to select a theoretical strategy and continue the work of developing and validating new nursing diagnoses. Derdiarian (1988) proposed that practicing nurses should be taught to formulate, test, and evaluate new nursing diagnoses (p. 139). Gebbie and Lavin claim that

> There is no category here that might not be rejected by nurses at a second or subsequent conferences, nor is there any claim that these categories cover the entire domain of nursing. Any rejection should be based on clinical evidence that the diagnosis provides no basis for nursing intervention. (1975, pp. 57–58)

Carpenito (1993) disagrees, saying that nurses should be spending more research time on the diagnoses that already exist, not on making new ones.

Submission guidelines were revised and published in the proceedings of the ninth conference. Considering the amount of work involved in the submission procedure, it seems highly unlikely that practicing nurses could undertake this task. Furthermore, the acceptance and placement of a diagnosis into the taxonomy is done by the Taxonomy Committee and is not open to scrutiny by the General Assembly. Porter (1986) notes that this procedure is in contrast to accepted taxonomic science, because the general membership does not have the final vote. Avant, on the other hand, maintains that voting is "unwise and scientifically unsound as a method of choosing" (1990, p. 54) and recommends that teams of scientists and clinicians make decisions regarding the presentation of adequate evidence for a nursing diagnosis. It was unclear how disagreements between the members of such teams would be handled.

RULES OF EVIDENCE

After a diagnosis is recognized as worthy of consideration, it is subjected to the rules of evidence specified by the discourse in order to determine approval and integration into the grid of specification. The 1982 guidelines consisted of the following five sections of information required for consideration:

A. *The category label (or title)*. In this section, applicants were asked to identify how the "label refers to an identifiable clinical entity."
B. *Common etiological factors*. This section required the identification of the etiological subcategory.
C. *The defining characteristics of the diagnostic category*. These were to be the "observable signs and symptoms that are present when the health problem is present."
D. *Supporting materials*. This category consisted of literature to support the category label, the etiological categories, and the defining characteristics.

E. *Rating of independent nursing involved in treating the health problem.* The rating in this category was to be identified as high, medium, or low, depending on degree of independent nursing therapy commonly involved in treating the diagnosis (Gordon, 1982b, pp. 340–341).

The term *accepted nursing diagnosis* was defined specifically at the fourth national conference (Kim & Moritz, 1982) as that which is, "in the opinion of the National Group, a health problem amenable to nursing intervention which has been sufficiently defined for clinical testing" (p. 6).

The submission guidelines were refined and published again in the proceedings of the seventh conference (McLane, 1987). E*tiology* was changed to defining characteristics, major and minor, and supplemental information became optional (McLane, 1987). Another revision took place at the ninth conference, which required a new diagnosis to be submitted complete with a label, a definition, defining characteristics, related factors, and literature/clinical validation support (Carroll-Johnson, 1991). A list of "To-Be-Developed Diagnostic Concepts and Definitions" were published in McFarland and McFarlane (1993) and included diagnoses such as "Ineffective Management of Therapeutic Regimen (Families)" and "High Risk for Loneliness" (p. 766).

After a diagnosis was accepted, tested, and approved, it was placed into the taxonomic structure and was assigned a number with respect to its position in the structure of Human Response Patterns. For example, the diagnosis of Altered Protection is numbered 1.6.2.

GRID OF SPECIFICATION

Discourses identify defining characteristics, quantify definitions, arrange subjects in a taxonomy, attribute causal mechanisms, and give rules for the application of the subjects to individual bodies. The use of the phrase *grid of specification* emphasizes the process of constructing a taxonomy and applying the grid in practice situations. Once identified and accepted according to the rules of evidence, nursing diagnoses were integrated into a grid of specification. NANDA's Taxonomy I was a grid of specification because the taxonomy divided the diagnoses from each other, related them, and placed them under a classification scheme.

At the fifth conference, Webster (1984) presented a paper on classification schemes in science and recommended to the conference participants that nursing diagnoses remain an alphabetical listing at that point. He emphasized that since nurses deal with both the general and the specific, the most important point about the process of diagnosing was the manner in which the diagnosis was assigned to the patient (Webster, 1984, p. 24). From a Foucaultian perspective, however, grids of specification delimit the practice of the discipline. The grid is not a neutral tool; it structures the interventions. Arguing that the important issue is how a nurse uses a diagnosis ignores the process by which the reified concept of diagnosis defines the way the nurse functions in the clinical encounter.

At the first conference, it was evident to the participants that entities in classification systems were not supposed to overlap, and yet they recognized that some of the nursing diagnoses did just that. This overlap was attributed to lack of scientific knowledge and not to anything about the diagnostic entity or the classification scheme (Gebbie & Lavin, 1975, p. 59). This situation continued to be discussed as a problem at succeeding conferences. Kritek (1986), for example, suggested to the sixth conference that hierarchical, mutually exclusive sorts of classification schemes might be too limiting for the concepts of human responses, but the work on the previously described unitary man/human response pattern framework continued.

Work continued to expand the grid of specification beyond the diagnoses. McCloskey et al (1990) argued for standardized language about nursing treatments; the links among diagnoses, treatments, and outcomes; facilitation of the development of information systems and decision making; assistance in the determination of costs for nursing services and planning for resources; the provision of a language to communicate the unique functions of nursing; and articulation with classification systems of other health care providers. McCloskey & Bulechek (1993) then went on to expand the grid of specification to a taxonomy of nursing interventions.

THE DISAPPEARANCE OF SUBJECTS

Discourses contain rules for the appearance and the dismissal of subjects. Consider two examples of diagnoses that have been suggested as candidates for removal from the grid of specification.

Jenny (1987) argued that knowledge deficit was not a human response or a nursing diagnosis. By using the criteria of appropriate conceptual focus, necessary diagnostic attributes, theoretical validity, and clinical utility, she concluded that the diagnosis is not legitimate and suggested that it be dropped from the taxonomy. She argued that knowledge deficit is more properly a risk factor, contributing factor, etiological factor, or defining characteristic of some other diagnosis.

Pokorny (1985) agreed with Jenny and found no critical defining characteristic of the diagnosis of knowledge deficit, although the data suggested that an important indicator of the diagnosis was the patient's verbal statement of a need for information or clarification. Jenny argued that "the continued use of the diagnosis Knowledge Deficit perpetuates the false assumption that knowledge is the sole and/or automatic determinant of human behavior" (1987, p. 185).

Following Jenny's analysis, further clinical support for eliminating the nursing diagnosis of knowledge deficit was provided by Dennison and Keeling (1989). Based on clinical data, these authors concluded that knowledge deficit falls outside the boundaries of the discipline and that the label encourages nurses to focus attention on the promotion of knowledge as an entity rather than addressing a behavior related to the patient's lack of information (p. 142). Despite these arguments, knowledge deficit remained in the grid of specification, although it was recommended at the ninth conference that the diagnosis be either revised or deleted (Carroll-Johnson, 1991, p. 28).

As another example, consider the diagnosis of noncompliance. Keeling, Utz, Shusler, and Boyle (1993) argued that the diagnosis of noncompliance should be abandoned by NANDA. They reasoned that it is not congruent with nursing ethically, historically, or philosophically; has doubtful clinical utility; and is inherently pejorative. The authors suggested that the diagnosis of noncompliance should be replaced with a diagnosis phrased variously as "need for commitment to treatment, or inability to adapt to treatment regimen, or self-care deficit, or potential for client participation in cure" (p. 96). Despite such attempts, noncompliance also remained in the grid of specification.

The perseverance of diagnoses despite evidence that they do not meet NANDA's criteria for acceptability suggested that the discourse itself had attained a certain degree of authority within the discipline that conferred some degree of immunity to critique. The participation of the discourse in foundational science bestowed stability to the constructs that carried conceptual permanence with or without external justification. Scientific labeling is justification enough.

As an example of such conceptual momentum, consider that Carpenito (1993) argued that all clinical research should be framed in terms of nursing diagnosis. She justified this by saying that if a study is not phrased in terms of nursing diagnosis, all you have is a nice little story about nursing in your town, but if the language of nursing diagnosis is used, you are expanding nursing knowledge (Carpenito, 1993).

AUTHORITIES OF DELIMITATION

The process of applying the power/knowledge, or the practices, of the discourse is structured by the grid of specification. The diagnoses are applied to the individual bodies of nurses and patients in a time/space structured in part by authorities of delimitation. The authorities of delimitation are the disciplines that control the existence and limits of the space for the action of the discourse. In the case of nursing diagnosis, these authorities are largely physicians, hospital administrators, and insurance companies, because they determine the patient's entrance to the health care system. This entrance is also subject to the petition of an individual patient, family, or concerned other and is sometimes accomplished without the consent of the patient, such as in the case of some admissions to mental health facilities.

It is clear that the description of the clinical encounter by the discourse of nursing diagnosis was not an autonomous act, but the authorities of delimitation are unacknowledged in the discourse. The bodies to which we apply the discourse of nursing diagnosis are those identified by medicine in the case of the patient and by the education, licensing, and hiring criteria in the case of the nurse. The subdisciplines of nursing that do not fit this model exactly include public health and advanced practice nurses who provide primary care, for neither of these subdisciplines use nursing diagnosis.

HOW THE DISCOURSE IS USED ON THE BODIES OF PEOPLE

Once the authorities of delimitation identify the bodies to which the discourse is applied, there exist rules for the application of the diagnoses in the space/time of the clinical encounter. The truth claims of the discourse are applied to human bodies using the language of the discourse. In general, what happens in the clinical encounter was conceptualized by the 1980 ANA Social Policy Statement as follows: "A nurse's conceptualization or diagnosis of a presenting condition is a way of ascribing meaning to it" (p. 11).

Used in the clinical encounter, the act of ascribing meaning serves to constitute the individuals involved (in this case the nurse and the patient) for themselves and others in prescribed ways, according to the rules of the discourse. Ascribing meaning to a situation assumes that the situation had no meaning before the discourse described it. This action is an interested move of power, but discussions of interests and/or power are nowhere represented in the discourse.

Specifically, the diagnoses were used on the bodies of the nurse and patient to determine treatments and to predict outcomes. "Nursing diagnosis should devise a way to engineer the uncertainty out of patient care situations and thus minimize the number of incorrect inferences" (Shamansky & Yanni, 1983, p. 48; see also Kritek, 1985). Note that this quote uses the instrumental (or technical) word *engineer*.

The discourse specified the behavior of the nurse by prescribing the proper assessment procedures, the array of acceptable diagnoses, the interventions that were appropriate to the diagnoses, and the outcomes that indicate success. The discourse also specified the behavior of the patient by assuming compliance with the process of disclosing data to the nurse (confession) and by assigning outcome behaviors that were considered acceptable to nursing.

These specifications assumed a hierarchical power relation of the nurse as a social agent and the patient as the recipient of nursing care. This assumption of hierarchy was not referred to specifically, because science is assumed to be value-free and its application by social agents is not appropriately questioned by ethical discourse. The result was a technical, mechanical discourse of prediction and control of social effects consistent with current power relations, assumed to be for the good of patients but excluding their voice.

ACKNOWLEDGMENT OF INDIVIDUAL DIFFERENCES

It is instructive to note where individual differences, deviations, and complaints by patients were allowed to emerge in the discourse. From a foundational perspective, the diagnoses should be the names of real things in the real world that can be investigated in a scientific manner. The results of these investigations should provide universal knowledge that can be used by social agents, or trained professionals, to help people become more normal (whether they want to or not). In the continuing problem of reconciling general knowledge with clinical practice, the question of individual variations arose in the discourse of nursing diagnosis.

Individual patient differences were supposed to be acknowledged in the *due to* or *related to* part of the diagnostic statement (Carpenito, 1993; McFarland & McFarlane, 1993). The first half of the diagnostic statement was assumed to be universally applicable to all human beings because it was constructed using foundational science. The second half of the diagnostic statement contained the specific individual etiology. However, the possible etiologies were already spelled out in the handbooks and textbooks (Carpenito, 1984; McFarland & McFarlane, 1993).

The diagnoses were assigned by assessment using universal signs and symptoms, and the causal etiologies were assigned from the list of possible "individual" etiologies. The full nursing diagnosis statement can thus be viewed as an attempt to combine a universal scientific entity and an individual clinical situation in a unique classification (Taylor, 1979). One problem with the clinical application of generalized knowledge is that probability statements resulting from scientific studies describe not the tendencies of individuals but of groups.

Confusion regarding these dimensions of the concept of diagnosis was widespread. For example, consider Fitzpatrick's (1990) description of the axes considered for Taxonomy II that included age and chronicity. She argued that using axes will integrate the "clinical with the scientific for discipline development" (p. 106). Henderson defined nursing practice as consisting of "both nursing intervention based on nursing diagnosis and nursing care originating in patient problems or health problems" (1978, p. 79), which assumed that nursing diagnoses and patient problems are separate entities. Presumably, this combination was made in order to capture more of the individual patient's unique circumstances within a generalized system of unique nursing knowledge.

Confusion regarding this concept was further evident in the discussion concerning the "validity" of diagnoses for individual clients. Noting that the diagnoses were not always valid in clinical practice led to the foundational conclusion that the validity should be measured on a scale. What to do with cases of marginal validity was not addressed.

Derdiarian (1988) produced three methods for nurses to validate nursing diagnoses in practice situations with individual patients. One method was asking the patient if she or he agrees with the diagnosis. The second was checking with another nurse, and the third was using existing knowledge. Conceivably, these three approaches may yield conflicting answers, but this possibility also was not addressed.

Lunney (1990) also discussed what she called the "accuracy" of nursing diagnoses. Her study concluded that accuracy is complex and situational. She presented an ordinal scale of minus one to plus five to measure accuracy of a nursing diagnosis, and she assigned defining characteristics for each level of accuracy. Accuracy in this context is the measure of how well the nursing diagnosis fits the "real" situation in terms of a number. Like Derdiarian's method of checking "validity," Lunney's method attempted to combine a universally applicable scientific concept with an individual case, in order to determine some degree of truth or applicability measured on a scale. She did not address how to ascribe treatments to diagnoses that have varying degrees of validity.

Maas, Hardy, and Craft (1990) called this idea of accuracy, or validity, the relationship between the nurse's inferred problem and the patient's "true problem" (p. 25). The true problem was an entity assumed to exist in an objective manner separate from our understanding of. In other words, the *object* of the discourse, the human response, was a true problem, and the nurse's inferred problem was the subject of the discourse, the diagnosis. If the science was performed correctly, there would be perfect correspondence between the patient's true problem and the nurse's choice of diagnosis.

The manner in which individual differences among nurses and patients were treated can be described as normalization. Recall that the process of normalization involves the statistical average as defined by research. The statistical average becomes the standard to which individual cases are compared in the process of assessment (Carlson, Craft & McGuire, 1982). Interventions by social agents should then be applied to the bodies of the patients with the goal of producing more normal outcomes. For example, consider the following quote: "The client's/patient's health status is compared to the norm in order to determine if there is a deviation from the norm and the degree and direction of deviation" (American Nurses Association, 1973).

Interventions become a normalizing influence on nurses as well as patients—normalizing the nurse's behavior within the clinical encounter toward what has been scientifically determined by the discourse. Indeed, idiosyncratic diagnoses are discouraged. "Conference participants have at least implied that they do not wish to see nurse educators developing 'diagnoses for use in teaching' as a separate or primary task distinct from 'diagnoses for use in research', etc." (Gebbie, 1982, p. 11). The choice for the clinician became a choice concerning which of the standardized diagnoses complete with standardized interventions would be used.

For example, at the fifth conference, Roy (1984) argued that a nursing diagnosis taxonomy could and should serve as a guide for practice. In other words, the judgment of the nurse takes certain prescribed paths with respect to empirically demonstrated trajectories in order to meet desirable outcome criteria for a patient as the discourse has determined them to be. The ANA identified a critical task for the future of nursing as "the implementation of standards of practice through the development of criteria related to specific nursing diagnoses" (Phaneuf, 1985, p. 1). In effect, the practice of nursing, as well as the outcome of nursing, were to be judged by criteria from the normalizing discourse of nursing diagnosis.

To this end, Bulechek, Kraus, Wakefield, and Kowalski (1990) presented a guide to measure whether or not nursing diagnosis was being implemented in a satisfactory manner in a hospital practice environment. The authors concluded that certain elements of a model of professional practice had to be in place before nursing diagnosis could be successfully implemented. The list included the notions of self-governance, accountability, and direct access to clients for diagnosis and treatment (p. 20). This view ignored the power relations of the hospital environment in favor of the professional model of social agency as "service to humanity."

Like other discourses that participate in foundational assumptions, nursing diagnosis revealed itself to be a value-laden discourse. Normalization is a value assumed through participation in power/knowledge. The power relations inherent within the process of normalization are not changed by having the patient participate in goal setting or the planning of care because the diagnosis, interventions, and outcomes are already set, thereby severely limiting the available speaking positions. Patients and nurses have only the illusion of choices within present power relations supported by the discursive practices of the discourse.

Normalization, of course, has its sphere of useful applications. Indeed, there may be certain limited statements people can justifiably make about the normal physiology of a healing fractured femur. There are, however, more limited numbers of statements people can justifiably make about people who have fractured femurs. The further away the claims move from physiology, the more dependent on the social context the answers become.

WHAT GUIDES THE DISCOURSE

Conflicting goals seem to govern the appearance, disappearance, replacement, and coexistence of the theoretical strategies for the generation of a taxonomy. The conflict between theory development and practical application has been discussed. Another goal apparent in the discourse can be termed theory development for the purpose of control of clinical phenomena at the population level. Henderson, for example, asserted that nursing diagnoses were the first step in theory development "that can be used for prediction and control" (1978, p. 77).

Fawcett complained that pragmatic concerns seemed to be more important than theory development, saying that development "appears to have proceeded in a contextual vacuum and has many indications of continuing to be guided by pragmatic, rather than theoretical, interests" (1986, p. 397). This position assumed that theory provides context and that pragmatics do not. Fawcett argues,

> If nursing diagnosis is to become an integral and meaningful part of nursing science and nursing practice, then theoretical interests must guide future work. I believe that this will occur if further development of nursing diagnosis is clearly based on explicit assumptions that are part of a conceptual model of nursing. . . the work done by the nurse theorist group associated with NANDA appears to be a conceptual model reflecting their particular assumptions about nursing. Although they tried to fit the list of diagnoses to their model, the fit seems forced at best and illogical at worst. (1986, p. 397)

Meleis agreed with Fawcett, saying nursing diagnoses "do not emanate from a coherent theoretical perspective" (1991, p. 161).

Also agreeing with Fawcett, Logan & Jenny (1990) argued that nursing diagnoses were not amenable to independent nurse functions and that they would have to be rewritten to do so. Logan argued that nursing diagnoses should be limited to only independent nursing functions. These functions would be derived from theoretical abstractions of nursing phenomena and would be completely unrelated to the functions of other disciplines.

Others argued that the diagnoses should be generated from work in practice settings and not from conceptual frameworks. Serious questions were raised regarding the adaptation of theoretically generated diagnoses to clinical situations (Rasch, 1987). The taxonomy committee's plan to "generate recommendations for making the taxonomy functional in the service setting" did not happen (Kritek, 1984, cited by Porter, 1986). Gordon (1990), on the other hand, suggested that each diagnosis have its own separate conceptual theory base and clinical research.

Conflicting approaches also were evident in the construction of the taxonomy from the perspective of taxonomic science. Porter (1986) pointed out, for example, that it is logically unsound to use nine distinct taxonomic trees for nine overlapping concepts. These overlapping concepts were used as both an organizing principle and as separate taxons. Porter argues that despite the Taxonomy Committee's insistence that the approach was inductive, the resulting taxonomy was clearly created in a deductive manner (p. 138). Porter also noted that although the diagnoses were sorted into four levels of abstraction, according to taxonomic science, the entities that are classified by a taxonomy must all exist at the same level of abstraction in order for the organizing principles to sort them by similarities and differences (p. 137).

The assumptions underlying taxonomy development were clearly established. It is questionable to assume, for example, (1) that there are entities that nurses diagnose, (2) that diagnosis is an appropriate model for what it is that nurses do, (3) that it is a good thing for nurses to diagnose, (4) that a classification scheme can and should be developed, and (5) that discussions of power are not important.

ON THE AXIS OF AUTHORITY

The right to pronounce truth in the realm of the clinical encounter was claimed by NANDA on the basis of its imitation of the discourses of medicine and science within a linguistically constructed professional domain that was claimed to be uniquely nursing. Other possible claims to the power of pronouncing truth in the clinical encounter have failed. Levine (1989), for example, called the failure of the ANA's efforts to convene various groups with an interest in classification schemes for nursing diagnoses a defeat for what she called *true scholarship*. She further claimed this will serve to legitimize and perpetuate what she called a badly flawed system.

At the eighth conference, Lang and Gebbie (1989) reported on the joint venture of the ANA and NANDA toward a submission to the International Congress of Nursing (ICN). They reported on the working relationships between the two organizations by publishing the recommendations of the Collaborative Group on Taxonomies/Classifications of Nursing Diagnoses. The recommendations by this group included the recognition by ANA of the NANDA Taxonomy as the official ANA Taxonomy of Nursing Diagnoses and the suggestion that collaboration should continue on a formal level (p. 13). In effect, this move legitimized NANDA's Taxonomy and marginalized any other classification scheme. NANDA's right to pronounce truth was thus preserved.

SYSTEMS FOR EDUCATION, ADVANCEMENT, AND ASSOCIATION

NANDA, which was incorporated in 1985, was and is the source and authority for the discourse. A refereed journal dedicated to research concerning nursing diagnoses began in 1990. The structure of the association provides justification, legitimacy, authority, and social presence for the discourse in a manner consistent with other disciplines based on a model of professional power and privilege. According to Foucault, this process confers on the practitioners of the discipline the status of social agents of the modern form of power— biopower. One unintended consequence of this status is a commitment to maintaining the current power relations.

AVAILABLE AND UNAVAILABLE SPEAKING POSITIONS

The first conference acknowledged that the participants were an elite group and wondered about the acceptance of nursing diagnosis by the "average" nurse (Gebbie & Lavin, 1975, p. 35). This was also reflected in the proceedings of the third and fourth conferences, when Gebbie complained, "Many other nurses, apparently accepting a view of the world that is much more formalized and authoritarian, see 'membership' in the conferences as based on some authority" (p. 11). Gebbie reiterated that all nurses must be encouraged to test, develop, and submit new and revised nursing diagnoses (1982, p. 11).

Membership in NANDA is open to all nurses from all settings, but participation requires major effort on the part of a full-time practicing nurse. Indirectly, this selects nurses who have the time and money to travel and work on their own without being paid for it. Speaking positions, therefore, are limited by the criteria of membership and participation in NANDA.

Kritek complained that

> the critical component needed is the clear and dominant voice of the nurse in practice, the staff nurse. Currently, that voice is the most often silenced, the least often heard in nursing dialogue. The challenge to those who have voice is clear: to enable the voice of the staff nurse in this process. (1989, p. 11)

Meleis concurred, stating that nursing diagnoses "do not represent the majority of nurses who have been caring for clients and for communities for years and whose levels of expertise range from the novice to the expert, nor could they do that" (1991, p. 412). Kim and Moritz added, "Further dialogue between the practitioners and the theorists is essential, and continued input from concerned experts in the area should be made available for a successful finale" (1982, p. xix).

Gebbie (1982) wrote that practicing nurses should be encouraged to join NANDA and to participate in Taxonomy development, while she realized that this placed a financial and time burden on them. She also suggested that "At some point, it may be necessary to formalize some method of qualifying for participation to ensure that new people can bring new ideas and energy without causing undue delay" (p. 12).

Positions from which to speak this discourse were thus limited by the hegemonic dominance of NANDA. At the seventh conference business meeting, a motion was passed stating "that NANDA go on record as supporting the concept that only registered, professional nurses be responsible and accountable for identifying the nursing diagnoses for their patient population" (McLane, 1987, p. 529). One implication of this motion was that nurses who are not registered, or are not professional, have no right to wield this language. This restriction assumed a certain degree of power inherent in the discourse that needed to be limited to a certain speaking position as defined by NANDA. This motion also assumed that people who do not meet the speaking criteria should not enjoy this privilege of acting as a social agent. It is not clear how this was to be enforced, but it was clear that NANDA was the decision-making body for approving the use of nursing diagnoses.

PRESERVATION AND TRANSMISSION OF THE DISCOURSE

The discourse was and is preserved and transmitted in a manner that consolidates the dominance of NANDA as the pronouncer of truth. This is accomplished by NANDA publications, conference proceedings, newsletters, speakers' bureau, workshops developed by NANDA, and dissemination to faculty who teach the discourse to students. NANDA news and committee reports are included in the journal *Nursing Diagnosis*. Guidelines for conducting workshops were presented at the fourth conference (Kim & Moritz, 1982).

The discourse is thus disseminated in many ways. The ANA revised the Standards of Clinical Nursing Practice in 1991. The standards include competence as demonstrated by the nursing process, which includes diagnosis. Shoemaker (1989) argued that nursing diagnoses should be taught in graduate as well as undergraduate curricula. Lee and Strong (1985) used nursing diagnosis to assess competence in nursing of recent graduates, using Likert scale ratings by the graduates and their faculty. The American Association of Critical Care Nurses used nursing diagnosis as the framework for conceptualizing nursing practice in their outcome standards.

These structural mechanisms for the preservation and transmission of the discourse provide necessary justification for the acceptance and use of the discourse by practitioners within the clinical encounter. Having a history, an incorporated association complete with bylaws, a journal, and a national forum lends legitimacy to the discourse entirely apart from the content of the discourse.

HANDLING OF IMPERFECTIONS

Imperfections in the discourse of nursing diagnosis have been classed as major or minor, and approaches to handling them are based on assumptions concerning the underlying value of the discourse as a whole with respect to professional goals. Some authors have argued that acknowledged imperfections in construction, application, and dissemination of nursing diagnosis should be handled with more clinical research (Carpenito, 1993; Fawcett, 1986; Kritek, 1985). Others have viewed the imperfections as indicative of deeper problems that cannot be addressed by more research.

Shamansky and Yanni (1983), for example, provided a broad critical rejection of the discourse and concluded that nursing diagnosis should be abandoned. It is significant to note that they identified their article as a "minority opinion." The authors cited such difficulties as frequent disagreement between expert practitioners in their choice of diagnoses, decreased interdisciplinary communication, and lack of precise language that matches the clinical situation.

Kritek (1985), while refusing to identify herself as a "true believer in nursing diagnosis" (p. 3), agreed with some points about the weaknesses in the discourse as identified by Shamansky and Yanni. However, Kritek did not agree with Shamansky and Yanni that the difficulties they describe are indicative of overwhelming inadequacy. In Kritek's view, the selected imperfections do not support the case that the effort should be abandoned. Kritek maintains that a taxonomy is itself a self-correcting device for dealing with inconsistencies because of the scientific nature of taxonomies (1989, p. 9). This assumption of the value of scientific inquiry (in this case, taxonomic science) ignores the question of the appropriateness of the choice to develop a taxonomy in the first place.

Fredette made the point that imperfections in nursing diagnosis with respect to the notion of causality make it difficult for the practitioner to identify how to direct the plan of care (1988, p. 33). Fredette did not see this imperfection as a major problem, saying that the solution to this imperfection is further dialogue between the practical approach and the scientific approach. Imperfections in the discourse could certainly be addressed by the official organization, but the important point is that the power to do so resides with the association and not the clinicians.

NANDA does not pass official judgment on books about nursing diagnosis, but individuals review books and articles, and the reviews are published in the proceedings of the conferences. Other reviews of books are published in the journal *Nursing Diagnosis*. Imperfections can certainly be noted and judged in this manner, since these two sources are official publications that carry much weight. The power to pronounce truth is further consolidated in this process.

THE AXIS OF VALUE OR JUSTIFICATION

The technologies of power used in the discourse of nursing diagnosis have been overtly justified within the discourse by reference to nurse empowerment and improved patient outcomes. Carpenito (1993), for example, complained that some authors were against nursing diagnosis simply because they saw it only as a way to empower nurses, when in fact it benefits patients at the same time.

On a deeper level, the justification for the application of disciplinary technologies rests on the assumption, consistent with the notion of bio-power, that power/knowledge confers the status of social agency on its practitioners. It is then the responsibility of the social agents to apply the power/knowledge for the assumed benefit of those whose have been so constituted by the discourse itself, whether or not the patients believe this is the case. Disciplinary technologies assume that nurses are justified in deriving goals and interventions without full participation of patients (Allen, 1987b, p. 46). In other words, patients are specifically constituted by the discourse to be self-revealing targets of normalization strategies wielded by social agents. As social agents, nurses truly believe that they are advancing civilization by improving the lives of those people they have scientifically determined as needing the application of the power/knowledge that nurses alone possess.

At the first conference, it was stated that the diagnoses should be validated officially through the ANA or the National League for Nursing (NLN) (Gebbie & Lavin, 1975, p. 4). The conference organizers also sought approval from several nonnursing authorities—physicians, medical records librarians, the Joint Commission, and hospital administrators—by having representatives participate in a panel presentation to the conference (pp. 4–5). NANDA's authority has since grown to the point that external validation by other nursing authorities has become unnecessary. Spin-off discourses such as the discourse of nursing interventions demonstrate the power of NANDA.

Creason (1992) proposed the following patient clinical outcome criteria to answer the question of whether or not specific nursing diagnoses are justified:

1. Do they reflect what is actually happening with the patient? (validity)
2. Are they sufficiently defined so that any nurse observing the same cues would arrive at the same diagnosis? (reliability)
3. Are they useful in designing nursing interventions?
4. Do they clearly communicate the condition of the patient among nurses and the direction for nursing interventions?
5. Is each one sufficiently independent of the other to promote clarity?
6. Will the patient benefit?
7. Can they be used in conjunction with medical diagnoses?
8. What research base do we presently have to support them, and what further research is needed?

It is important to note that the following question was not asked: Do nurses have the power within the hospital environment to cause all of the criteria listed to happen or be measured?

These criteria reflect the justification of nurses as social agents. The language of foundational science assumes that description and action in new regions of experience is justified, because knowledge generation provides power over ignorance. Following the repressive hypothesis, knowledge generation is assumed to liberate people from the slavery of ignorance by the provision of knowledge without values. Using the language of science, nurses are therefore justified in their research on the "human responses to illness" or the "human responses to the human responses to illness" or any other region we would care to describe, as long as the carefully described territory does not encroach too much on the terrain of some other discipline. Such encroachment would be seen as resistance to current power relations and would create tension with other disciplines. So far, that has not happened between nursing and any other discipline.

Using the language of professionalism, we are justified in applying the knowledge we construct to our own bodies and the bodies of our patients by educating social agents in foundational science and professional behavior created discursively by our discourse. In the shifting web of power relations, social status can be embodied by emulating successful models in newly constructed social situations.

JUSTIFICATION FOR THE PUNISHMENT OF PARTICIPANTS

In order to consolidate the power/knowledge of the discipline embodied in the social agents, control is exercised over the participants in the discourse in the manner of the model of professionalism. The justification provided by nursing is the socially valued one of patient safety. As an example of such justified punishment, consider that Carpenito (1993) believes that missing a diagnosis in nursing should be considered malpractice in the same way as it is in medicine. This belief is congruent with the dominant discourse of nursing diagnosis, which is the discourse of medicine. This belief seems incongruent, however, with a nursing diagnosis of "effective breast feeding" or "functional grieving."

Since the ANA standards of nursing practice were based partially on the ability to make nursing diagnoses, it is conceivable that nurses could be sued or fired from their jobs for not doing so. Furthermore, the use of nursing diagnoses was meant to be a distinguishing feature of the differing levels of nursing practice at the first conference (Gebbie & Lavin, 1975, p. 26).

The systems for punishment of participants could thus be identified as the individual economic unit that hires the nurse, the association and law under which the nurse practices, and the educational institution in the case of the student. Correction, normalization, and punishment thus have systems in place for their application on the body of the nurse.

JUSTIFICATION FOR THE SUPPRESSION OF OTHER DISCOURSES

When a discourse gathers membership, influence, power, and momentum, seeking hegemony, creating definitions, and highlighting differences between itself and other competing discourses, it seeks to discredit and suppress other discourses in the interests of solidifying the ideology that constitutes meaning. The arguments in favor of nursing diagnosis gain force because of the general acceptance of the scientific and professional approaches highly valued in our culture. A dominant discourse, convinced of the "rightness" of the ideology, seeks to exclude other viewpoints in an effort to accrue power/knowledge by citing benefit to some group or another, who "don't know what is best for them."

The discourse of nursing diagnosis follows this model. For example, in 1987 the Journal of the Association of Operating Room Nurses (AORN) was asked to edit articles and use the term *nursing diagnosis* only for official NANDA diagnoses. The editors refused, saying nurses make diagnoses that are not NANDA ones all the time (Puterbaugh, Koralewski, & Falkenhagen, 1987).

Harrington proposed that educators should limit teaching diagnoses to the NANDA list only, saying "random creative efforts in the area of nursing diagnosis threaten the society of nursing and the development of a taxonomy" (1988, p. 94). All communication in the discourse, in her view, should be channeled through NANDA.

> Educators have the responsibility to control the channels of communication so that responses are productive. . . . Students should not be confused, and they should not add to the confusion, by using creative, personal, and non-communicable diagnoses. If they all use different languages, students graduating from nursing schools across the country will not be able to communicate with one another about nursing diagnosis. (Harrington, 1988, p. 94)

These examples demonstrate the strong influence of NANDA with respect to the suppression of other discourses. The fervor apparent in quotes from Harrington show personal commitment to a "cause" that seems phrased in the same way as a political movement. A similarity between proponents of nursing diagnosis and proponents of a religion has been noted before (Kritek, 1985).

THE INFLUENCE OF THE DISCOURSE OF MEDICINE

This section will present evidence that the dominant influence on the internal structure of the discourse of nursing diagnosis is medicine. Whether the intent of the text is to highlight the differences or the similarities between nursing and medicine, the language remains medical. In order to highlight the similarities and the differences at the same time, the medical language remains the basis of comparison. Like medicine, nurses diagnose, treat, and measure outcomes. Unlike medicine, nurses diagnose and treat human response patterns based on their own body of knowledge. Throughout this process, medicine is the privileged other, the invisible binary partner of nursing in the relation that defines nursing as a discipline. The following reasons support the claim that the dominant regularity in the discourse of nursing diagnosis is medicine:

1. *Word choice.* Recall that the act of definition is a move of power. The choice of the word *diagnosis* at the first conference maintains both the similarities and differences between nursing and medicine at the same time, without

challenging the status quo of power and influence. As we have seen, this approach is assumed to be justified by the adoption of the models of science, medicine, and professionalism.

Language is a very political and power-oriented activity (Levine, 1989). In the proceedings of the third and fourth conferences, it was speculated that the reason studies making use of nursing diagnosis were not being funded was that there was a "certain uneasiness with the use of the word 'diagnosis'. There are fears of what that evokes in other disciplines" (Kim & Moritz, 1982, p. 13). Levine (1966) had constructed the term *trophicognosis* to be used instead of *nursing diagnosis*, but this term never became popular. The influence of the discourse of patient needs and problems that was reflected in early definitions of nursing diagnosis has also faded. Despite opposition, the word *diagnosis* was adopted.

The derivations of definitions provided for nursing diagnosis are all medical. Derdiarian (1988) derived her definition of nursing diagnosis based on three different definitions of the word *diagnosis* from three different medical sources, which were then "adapted to nursing" (p. 138). Carlson and her colleagues (1982) based their definition on one of the three different components to the definition of *diagnosis* from *Webster's Dictionary*.

The words *treatment* and *intervention* are also widely represented. Gebbie (in Carlson et al., 1982) stated that "more nurses have come to describe their professional responsibility as the process of diagnosing and treating client conditions" (p. vii). Turkoski (1988) notes that the discourse of nursing diagnosis frequently uses medical diagnoses as descriptors (p. 143), medical labels, language, and models within the concept and design of the discourse (p. 144). The conspicuous absence of the word *disease* is noteworthy. Emphasis on the word *diagnosis* coupled with strict avoidance of the word *disease* reinforces the definition of nurses as "not-doctors." This approach uses imitation of the process while carefully avoiding turf battles.

The arguments involved in defining what it is that nurses diagnose assume that the applicability of the concept of diagnosis to nursing is already established. This assumption thereby diverts attention from the underlying question of whether or not nurses diagnose to the question of what it is that nurses diagnose.

The choice of classifying nursing diagnoses also reflects the medical discourse. The grid of specification, or the taxonomy, of nursing diagnosis was meant to mesh with existing classification schemes. Gebbie (1989) described and summarized the major classification systems in health care as the International Classification of Diseases, (ICD), the Common Procedural Terminology (CPT) in medicine, the Diagnostics & Statistics Manual (DSM) in the American Psychological Association (APA), the Systematized Nomenclature of Pathology (SNOP) in pathology, and the Systematized Nomenclature of Medicine (SNOMED) in medicine. She argued that any classification system in nursing must be translatable into currently existing coding schemes. "Anyone wishing to add or to replace a coding system in use will have to demonstrate both the need for and efficacy of the changes" (p. 49).

2. *The discourse is based on a model of symptomatology and etiology.* At the first conference, the diagnoses were referred to as having definitions that would be defined operationally in terms of "signs and symptoms," for example, the signs and symptoms of "incomplete grieving" (Gebbie & Lavin, 1975, p. 25). Gordon (1976) also explains "defining characteristics" of nursing diagnoses in terms of signs and symptoms. One reason cited for the importance of developing a classification system for nursing diagnosis is that it "allows application of epidemiological principles and methods to clinical nursing" (Carlson et al., 1982, p. 25). Carpenito (1983) uses the term *etiological factors*. At the seventh conference, Fitzpatrick (1987) advocated using the term *influencing factors* instead of etiology (p. 63).

McFarland and McFarlane (1993) also use the word *symptoms* for the concept of defining characteristics of nursing diagnoses. For example, one diagnosis to be made and treated by nurses is "Altered Health Maintenance related to inability to secure adequate permanent housing for self and family" (McFarland & McFarlane, 1993, p. 23). One defining characteristic, or symptom, of this condition is *verbalization of inaccurate information*. Viewing verbalization of inaccurate information as a symptom of "Altered Health Maintenance related to inability to secure adequate permanent housing for self and family" is a good example of the pathologizing of everyday life.

McFarland and McFarlane (1993) also use the concept of *risk factors* in their presentation of some diagnoses stated as "high risk." Assessment of risk factors, as well as signs and symptoms, became an important component of identifying nursing diagnoses. For example, the risk factors for "high risk for activity intolerance" include sedentary lifestyle, chronic or progressive disease, fatigue or weakness, deconditioned status, weight more than 15% over acceptable standard, pain, and refusal to participate in prescribed activities.

Use of the term *risk factors* also demonstrates an emphasis on epidemiology and population-based statistics. At the fifth national conference, Toth (1984) praised nursing diagnosis for the opportunity to compare patients classed as "acute diabetic patients who are non-compliant with therapy because of a knowledge deficit" from one hospital to another, statistically in terms of their length of stay (p. 100). Population-based diagnoses are thus justified, and the noncompliant label follows individual patients from one hospital to another. The potential for oppression will be discussed in the power analytic.

3. *The discourse emphasizes pathology.* Fawcett (1990) argued specifically against what she called "the fact" that NANDA's system is based on an externally driven biomedical perspective with an emphasis on pathology. Fawcett argued that this biomedical perspective was inappropriate and should be replaced with a nursing perspective derived from a conceptual work by nursing theorists.

Pathology is also emphasized by the choice of the word *deficit*. NANDA diagnoses name states of deficit, impairment, and disturbance (Gordon, 1982a) and alterations in functions or in functional patterns (Pridham & Schutz, 1985). Diers (1986) points out that the word *deficit* implies defect. She questions certain uses of the word *deficit* in the discourse of nursing diagnosis, such as *knowledge deficit*, and asks how it is that knowledge can be defective.

The overwhelming emphasis on pathology is brought into sharp contrast by the inclusion of *diagnoses* that are health related. Such a diagnosis is that of "Effective Breast-feeding" (McFarland & McFarlane, 1993). Popkess-Vawter (1991) recommends adding more wellness-related diagnoses, such as functional grieving, adequate individual coping, improved coping, activity tolerance, and effective airway clearance (p. 22). The placement of wellness-related diagnoses in the taxonomy is unclear. States of health becoming a diagnosis are consistent with the medicalization of everyday life in the era of managed care as discussed in chapter 1.

4. *The discourse emphasizes a disease model* (Meleis, 1991). The ICD was one of the classification schemes studied at the first conference. It was suggested at that conference that the medical classification of diseases (SNOMED, or Systematized Nomenclature of Medicine) was the only one that had room in its numerical classification system for nursing diagnoses to be added (Gebbie and Lavin, 1975, p. 20). Since NANDA was denied inclusion in the International Classification of Diseases (Webb, 1992), Clark and Lang (1992) recommend for nursing practice a separate international classification whose primary components are patients' needs, nursing actions, and patient outcomes.

5. *The discourse of nursing diagnosis has a strong physiological bias* (Webb, 1992). At the first conference, working groups were designated and assigned to a physiological system, even though the conference organizers record opposition to such a move as committing the system "irretrievably" to a pathological and disease-based model (Gebbie & Lavin, 1975, p. 5). The resulting diagnoses, predictably, reflect the organization of the working groups.

Approximately half of the diagnoses in Taxonomy I are physiologically based (Fitzpatrick et al., 1989). Carpenito (1993) is opposed to calling some of these physiological phenomena nursing diagnoses because she states that doing so takes on an accountability that is medical rather than not nursing. She also records that critical care nurses complain about the lack of physiological nursing diagnoses. Carpenito calls these diagnoses collaborative problems and complains that critical care nurses in general emphasize the collaborative problems in order to avoid dealing with the human response problems. Kritek (1985) argues that the only alternative to nursing diagnoses is "regressive adaptation to a medical paradigm" (p. 4). For critical care nurses, however, the "so-called medical model of treating anaphylactic shock better describes what we do for a patient than 20 different nursing diagnoses" (Curry, 1991, p. 124).

At the ninth conference, during the discussion of the work towards Taxonomy II, critical care nurses became dismayed at the deletion of physiological diagnoses that they felt were useful in their practice (Carroll-Johnson, 1991,

p. 51). The answer given by the committee working on Taxonomy II was that these diagnoses were still approved; since they did not represent independent nursing judgments, however, they did not fit within the new work on Taxonomy II and had been left out. The critical care nurses had been emphasizing the similarities of their practice and that of medicine, but the work on Taxonomy II emphasized the differences while still using the physiological language of diagnosis.

6. *The diagnoses are supposed to be applied in nursing practice in clinical situations, even though many nursing diagnoses do not seem to fit patient situations* (Frank, 1990). The diagnosis is established through the clinical judgment of the nurse, based on scientifically derived categories and recognition of symptoms and risk factors. The knowledge to diagnose and treat the problem that is constructed by the discourse is assumed to exist within the nurse by virtue of education and experience.

THE INFLUENCE OF THE DISCOURSE OF EMPIRICAL ANALYTIC SCIENCE

The discourse of medicine is based on empirical analytic science with foundational assumptions. Although diseases are historical constructs, they are regarded within the discourse of medicine as entities that exist apart from the medical conceptualization of them. Nursing diagnosis emulates medicine's participation in foundational science.

Recall that the assumptions of a foundational view of science include the existence of a foundation of absolutely true facts and the value-free nature of scientific activity (Hekman, 1986). The adoption of an unexamined medical model into the nursing model of diagnosis perpetuates the assumption that human problems are justifiably viewed as reified entities rather than social judgments.

Most nursing researchers are committed to the dominant empirical analytic paradigm as a model for the profession, and not only as a tool to answer appropriate questions (Dickson, 1993). Carpenito (1993) insisted that one of "nursing's problems" is that nurses have been content to be described by what they do, not by what they know. Carpenito holds that technicians are defined by what they do, and scientists by what they know (p. 92). Curtin (1978) argues, on the other hand, that nursing should be defined by its philosophy, not its functions. This debate between knowing and doing reflects the social value placed on knowledge over practice. Evidence that the discourse of nursing diagnosis is based on the assumptions of the empirical analytic foundational position is placed into the following categories:

1. *Reductionism.* The discourse of nursing diagnosis is based on a reductionist assumption (Tierney, 1987). The assumption is that the conceptualization

of human beings can be "reduced" to sets of diagnoses for ease of identification, treatment, and measurement of uniquely nursing outcomes. Doing so avoids the messy world of social context and value judgments. The reductionist perspective is valued in nursing diagnosis because of its perceived scientific, value-free nature.

For example, Gordon reported that some people were of the opinion that the classification scheme for nursing diagnoses, being reductionist, did not adequately reflect the holistic nature of nursing practice (1982a, p. 40). Kim (1983) added that nursing diagnoses are created entities that conflict with the concept of the "wholeness" of individual people (p. 139). Kritek, however, saw nursing diagnosis as "the point where holistic synthesis occurs" (1978, p. 40). Many patient experiences defy classification in NANDA terms (Pridham & Schutz, 1985).

Meleis called the diagnoses "esoteric in language and nonrepresentative of the complexity of human beings" (1991, p. 161). "There is a growing number of nurses who view the labeling inherent in the diagnostic process as too restrictive for describing human beings" (Mitchell & Santopinto, 1988, p. 25). Eleven years after Gordon's book, McFarland and McFarlane (1993) did not refer to holism at all; for them the term *wholeness* refers only to a notion of spirituality. Various authors have noted the lack of fit between Taxonomy I and the concept of unitary humans derived from the work of Martha Rogers, which was used as the organizing framework for the classification (England, 1989; Gordon, 1987; Roy, 1984; Smith, 1988).

2. *Determinism*. A strictly deterministic, linear view of causality is assumed by the discourse (Turkoski, 1988). Multiple causal factors are assumed to be discoverable and specifiable in advance (Bircher, 1986; Gordon, 1982a; Fitzpatrick, 1987; Forsyth, 1984). Nursing care is defined as effective when measurable, expected outcomes result from the planned action within the clinical encounter (McFarland and McFarlane, 1993). The deterministic view of human beings assumed by the discourse of nursing diagnosis has serious implications for nursing practice because it reflects nursing's commitment to empirical analytic science as the best criterion for a professional discipline (Allen, 1987b).

The emphasis on prediction reflects the linear view of causality. Carpenito (1993) claims that nursing diagnosis provides predictive scientific nursing care; "That is, we know in advance what a patient will probably need" (p. 94). According to Kritek, "Once we isolate phenomena, we can describe them, manipulate them, and create preferred outcomes; then we can have the effect we wish to have" (1985, p. 6). "Theory supporting nursing diagnosis must account for description, explanation, prediction and control of phenomena that nurses autonomously treat" (Wooldridge et al., 1993, p. 50).

Determinism is clearly reflected in Forsyth's presentation to the fifth conference, in which he states that although we cannot demonstrate the empirical existence of causality, we may indeed speak of correlations, associations, and relationships among the entities being observed (1984, p. 71). The assumption of causality from correlations, associations, and relationships is not statistically warranted. These descriptions assume that the phenomena we deal with can be isolated, identified, studied, and elicited without regard for the social context of the patient.

3. *Essentialism* (Allman, 1992; Dickson, 1993). Essentialism refers to the discredited assumption that words are names of unique things in a real world and that proper use of a word requires there being some invariant core set of properties that justify application of the word. The essentialist perspective has serious implications in nursing, not the least of which exists within the discourse of nursing diagnosis (see Allen, 1986; Thompson, 1992).

At the sixth conference, Kritek emphasized that taxonomic ordering should reveal the essential properties of phenomena (1986, p. 23). In Webster's (1984) paper, he discussed essentialism, recommending to the participants at the fifth conference that, given a choice between an essentialist view of empirical phenomena and the view that classification schemes reflect only our own conventions and not the nature of the phenomena of concern, "Wisdom seems to dictate some sort of intermediate position" (p. 21). Neither the wisdom nor the intermediate position was further described.

Porter (1986, p. 136) used Fleishman's (1982) definition of taxonomy as "the science of identifying and classifying entities, the study of the bases, principles, procedures and rules that enable classification" and asserts that a taxonomy is necessarily an essentializing discourse. Nonessentialist taxonomies would function by stipulative definitions, the measures of which are pragmatic and functional rather than essentialist (Allen, 1986). Recognition of the critique of essentialism is reflected in Kerr's presentation to the ninth national conference in which she states, "The essence of an element is not constant" (1991, p. 7). Kerr therefore describes methods for validation of diagnoses that include qualitative analysis along with cluster analysis, discriminant analysis, and fuzzy set methods (p. 12).

Some potential pitfalls of essentialist taxonomy development were pointed out at the first conference, including the danger of vague and/or overlapping categories and the logical possibility that nursing phenomena may not be amenable to standardization in an essentializing way (Gebbie & Lavin, 1975, p. 14).

Essentialism was reflected in the presentations to several conferences on taxonomic science (Bircher, 1986, p. 76; Gebbie & Lavin, 1975). Gebbie & Lavin (1975) emphasized that a taxonomy will order phenomena in ways that will reveal "essential properties and their relationships" (p. 13). On the other hand, Diers (1986) warned that the scientific assumption that "operational definitions" will name the essential properties of "vague" nursing diagnoses may be unwarranted.

According to Fleishman (1982), the purpose of using a taxonomic structure to categorize entities is to explain, in a causal way, why they have the properties they do and why they are similar and different from other entities in the structure. Porter (1986) added that a process or state cannot be a taxon, according to taxonomic science. The term *alterations*, for example, has been defined by NANDA as "the process or state of becoming or being made different without changing into something else" (McLane, 1987, Taxonomy I).

The influence of essentialism can also be seen in the emphasis on defining the unique characteristics of nursing itself. Nursing diagnosis often has been cited as the unique essential criterion for nursing as a discipline. Kritek claims that the"generation and classification of nursing diagnoses aims to clarify nursing's separate sphere and articulate those responsibilities that are uniquely nursing's. . . . Equality, even equity, requires a distinct domain to bring to the enterprise. . . . Certainly nursing diagnoses should enhance, not preclude collaboration" (1985, p. 4). If nursing were truly autonomous, then the nursing diagnosis would be as informative and useful to the physician as the medical diagnosis is to the nurse (Levine, 1989). Logan & Jenny (1990) proposed that nursing diagnoses address only independent nursing functions. In 1989, the ANA stated, "Until nurses can name what they do and assign a computer code to that name, we may be neither reimbursed nor recognized as a profession with unique skills and knowledge" (p. 3).

4. *The reification of entities.* Reification is the transformation of social relations from relations between persons to relations between things (Hiraki, 1992, p. 131). We refer to the individual "having" the diagnosis. The objects of the discourse, the human responses, are not viewed as social constructions. Kritek (1989) referred to this depersonalizing effect as a "challenge" for the language of nursing diagnosis, and Lindsay (1990) felt that human responses are real physical things. Quoting Watson (1990), Hiraki stated that the development of nursing knowledge that encourages the view of humans and health caring processes as problems to diagnose gives power to the problems and processes by according them law-like status, separated from the experiences of human beings (Hiraki, 1992, p. 19).

Reification assumes value-neutrality, and NANDA conferences assume the value-neutrality of nursing diagnoses as scientific concepts. Bircher (1986) told the sixth national conference that "nursing diagnosis is an abstract concept, an intellectual tool which is neutral. It is as powerful and constructive, or as weak and destructive, as the extent to which it is used appropriately and effectively toward the achievement of an end" (p. 73). On the contrary, according to Foucault, any technology is not neutral. Any disciplinary technology has unintended consequences with regard to the relationships between people. As stated by Hagey and McDonough, "Either supporters of nursing diagnosis see the categories as harmless without social context or they take as self-evident and acceptable the political outcomes such categories produce" (1984, p. 153). Tools structure their own use in discoverable ways. The power implications of reification are significant. Implications for oppression of patients and nurses will be addressed in the power analytic.

5. *The discourse of nursing diagnosis is based on instrumental knowledge.* This is a "formula approach to people, objectifying, codifying, and reifying human experiences with 'official knowledge' that takes on a life of its own; a life that is separate and decontextualized rather than connected" (Watson, 1990, quoted in Hiraki, 1992, p. 19).

For example, at the seventh conference, Levine raised what she called a "serious philosophical issue" with respect to the idea that the essence of nursing is treating human responses (1987, p. 51). She argued that this view assumes that humans are simply responding dependent systems, or "targets" for interventions without any consideration of a concept of human agency (p. 52).

6. *It holds natural science as the ideal* (Dickson, 1993; Donaldson & Crowley, 1978; Jacobs & Huether, 1978; Kim, 1983; Silva & Rothbart, 1984; Street, 1992; Thompson, 1985). Schilder and Edwards (1993), for example, argued that nursing researchers have been most concerned only with whether or not and to what extent their results are generalizable. Maas and her colleagues argued for strictly empirical methodological limitations on nursing diagnosis research "in order to get more funding and exposure in 'the scientific arena'" (1990, p. 30).

The ideal of natural science is reflected in the choice of the words and procedures of taxonomic science. For example, Kritek (1985) suggested that it might take nursing 300 years to complete the taxonomic system, if we consider the taxonomic development of the periodic table of elements. Even then, no classification system is ever complete (Harrington, 1988).

The ideal of natural science is also clearly represented in the comparisons made between nursing and other disciplines. Kritek (1985) compares nursing to quantum theory of physics, chemistry, behavioral sciences, and social sciences. Carpenito (1993) compares the diagnosis of decisional conflict to the diagnosis of pancreatitis because she argues that they are both objective entities scientifically describable and amenable to standardized treatments that professionals should be accountable for treating.

Natural science as the ideal is reflected in the "naturalism" of nursing diagnosis in the same manner as it is in the discourse of medicine (Allman, 1992). The assumptions of naturalism include the existence of an objective "nature" that is separate from human knowledge of it. Nature is assumed to exist prior to culture and social order. Knowledge and truth are therefore assumed to exist separately from power and morality (Allman, 1992). The discourse of nursing diagnosis treats the categories of the human responses (the objects of the discourse) as natural and universal scientific entities.

Natural science is also reflected in the style of statements because almost all of the diagnoses are phrased in terms of quantitative, foundational science. Two examples that represent the generation of a new nursing diagnosis using a qualitative methodology are Clunn (1984) and Logan and Jenny (1990). Qualitative research was, however, suggested at the ninth conference as one promising method for research in nursing diagnosis (Carroll-Johnson, 1991). Natural science is also reflected in the regularity that governs the style of the theoretical strategies (Tinkle & Beaton, 1983) used by the discourse to construct knowledge.

For example, at the first conference both inductive and deductive scientific strategies for the development of a taxonomy were suggested (Gebbie & Lavin, 1975, pp. 37–56). Among the deductive approaches suggested were Maslow's hierarchy of needs and various nursing theories that were current at the time (Gebbie & Lavin, 1975). It was suggested that since both the deductive and inductive strategies contain the possibility of error, one should not be picked over the other (Gebbie & Lavin, 1975, p. 56).

The debate concerning the inductive and deductive approaches has been given considerable attention. McCloskey (1987) presented the argument that Taxonomy I was created inductively, from concrete to abstract. Although Kim and Moritz (1982) argued that the products of the first two conferences (inductive) and the nurse theorists' work at the third and fourth conferences (deductive) might continue to run parallel (p. 7), they hoped the strategies would converge (p. 131). In the same volume of the proceedings of the third and fourth conferences, Gebbie stated that a specific decision was made in favor of the inductive approach at the first conference, but that this decision was proving very frustrating to the nurse theorists (1982, p. 9).

Kim (1983) took the position that NANDA, by adopting the inductive method, completely bypassed the question of a specific theoretical orientation for the classification system (the adoption of a framework called "unitary man" notwithstanding). She argued that the attempt to remain atheoretical by giving operational definitions, etiologies, and defining characteristics resulted in a multitheoretical framework instead (p. 140).

7. *It is a standardized model based on standards constructed from foundational science.* As such, it was assumed that the model could substitute for knowledge and experience in a novice situation and therefore could be a teaching guide. Concepts that are hard to measure were left out, causing items like caring and sensitivity to be devalued and/or not evaluated at all (Gordon, 1984). According to some authors, care based on predetermined standards contributes to the failure of treating persons as individuals (Bond, 1988; Niziolek & Shaw, 1991).

It is not clear whether a label from a standardized body of knowledge applied to specific human-environment interactions can be the empirical basis of nursing interventions. It is also not clear whether such labels can undergo taxonomic classification (Porter, 1986, p. 138). Standardized labels in clinical situations are barriers to practice because they limit creativity and individuality. In fact, a computerized nursing diagnosis system has been suggested: "The standardized language can be computerized and linkages between diagnoses, interventions, and outcomes can be discovered through documentation and study of actual patient care" (Bulechek & McCloskey, 1990, p. 27). Software would accept the patient data, produce diagnoses and the associated treatments, and become part of the patient's hospital record (Hirsch & Chang, 1990).

Harvey (1993) demonstrated that an ART-2 neural network agreed with expert nurses in the determination of nursing diagnoses. In a 1979 study, however, Matthews and Gaul found no relationship between the ability to make nursing diagnoses and critical thinking ability in both undergraduate students and graduate students. Assigning a diagnosis on the basis of clinical data does not, apparently, involve critical reasoning. Booth saw only one problem with a standardized language: nurses would lose track of patients' needs because of "laziness or being pressed for time" (1992, p. 33).

THE INFLUENCE OF THE DISCOURSE OF PROFESSIONALISM

Nursing, in imitation of the medical model, participates in, reinforces, and reflects the discourse of professionalism in U.S. culture. Medicine is generally considered the prototype model of a profession. In Foucaultian terms, it provides a normative view of reality, discourages and co-opts alternatives, absorbs their ideology, and has the social power to medicalize aspects of everyday life that have not been thought of as medical before, such as social role dysfunctions. The status and power of medicine is increased by an alliance with natural sciences because this allows the discourse to deny the ideological nature of its own knowledge (Street, 1992), even though medical knowledge is used in a clinical situation that includes many ideological components.

Nursing diagnosis participates in the discourse of professionalism because science and professional are believed to be co-extensive discourses (Dickson, 1993). For example, Carlson, Craft, and McGuire stated that the nursing diagnosis movement would result in greater professionalism for nurses (1982, p. x). According to Gebbie and Lavin, it had become necessary to "state . . . the reasons that some persons were receiving care from two professionals, the nurse asserting that they were seeing the patients for different problems than the physician" (1975, p. 1) In addition, they felt that "without such a system nurses will continue to experience difficulty in educating beginning practitioners, designing and performing research, and communicating nursing care within the nursing profession or across the health system" (p. 1).

At the third conference, Gebbie stated that "Movement on the classification is linked with movement toward professional and scientific maturity, and each feeds on the other" (1982, p. 12) and that the "long-term goal is to become a full profession" (p. 13). Carpenito (1993) specifically equated scientific with professional. Toth (1984) and Roberts (1990) even went so far as to advocate for the concept of "nursing DRG's" (Diagnostic Related Groups) for professional power and autonomy, and Roberts proposed to discuss "how nursing diagnosis can be used to achieve professional autonomy" (1990, p. 54). At the seventh conference, however, Gebbie warned that patterning fee schedules based on the medical model of payment (DRG's) reflected superficial imitation without true change: "It is as if we will 'get there' wherever that is, when we are paid just like 'them' " (1987, p. 39). She worried about superficially adopting a jargon that did not reflect any change in actual practice.

Turkoski (1988) analyzed the literature on nursing diagnosis from 1950 to 1985 and concluded that the relationship between professionalism and nursing diagnosis was not clear. As analyzed by Turkoski, two conflicting positions were represented in these works. The first position is that nursing diagnosis was instrumental in developing the concept of nursing as a profession. The second position consists of the belief that the professionalization of nursing has created the necessity for a specific nursing language. Turkoski concluded that these two positions continue to inform the discourse without resolution.

In Foucaultian terms, the discourse of nursing diagnosis participates in the expanding power/knowledge base over the details of everyday human life. The discourse of nursing diagnosis, by adopting the models of medicine, foundational science, and professionalism, participates in the processes of normalization, confession to social agents, and the medicalization and clinicalization of everyday life.

POWER ANALYTIC

This section presents an analysis of the web of power relations in which the discourse of nursing diagnosis is situated.

Domination of Patients

The domination of patients by nurses is extended by the discourse of nursing diagnosis by incorporating the unacknowledged assumption of elitism within the practice of nursing. The clinical encounter viewed from the discourse of nursing diagnosis is based on a model of social hierarchy and power.

The model of social agency assumed by the discourse of nursing diagnosis constitutes nurses as the authorities to deliver what the discipline decides is needed, not what the patient wants (Porter, 1992). Social agents have the duty of monitoring and upholding the status quo of power relations (Foucault, 1988) or risk being seen as unfaithful to their education and their science. This duty is clearly reflected in the goal of nursing to facilitate the patient's adaptation to current circumstances, whatever they are. Normal patient roles are described, defined, assessed, and treated by the social agent on the basis of clearly prescribed professional procedures.

Words modeled after medicine (such as *nursing diagnosis*) have unintended consequences that also increase nurses' domination over patients. Hiraki (1992) argued that when the empirical analytic tradition oversteps its bounds and becomes a metaphor for the entirety of nursing care, as it does within the discourse of nursing diagnosis, it reframes (re-creates, reconstructs) the reality of the clinical encounter in particular ways nurses might not have intended. "The nursing process is a problem solving method, and when it is inappropriately applied, has the power to decontextualize the nurse-patient relationship, work as a tool of institutional control, and perpetuate a technocratic ideology that is patriarchal in nature" (Hiraki, 1992, p. 129). This technocratic ideology constitutes patients as systems to be manipulated.

Domination of patients is also perpetuated by the control-based language of science. Wright and Levac (1992), for example, following Chilean biologist Maturana, argued that discourse based on "descriptions of truth" is an act of violence, defined as "holding one's opinion to be true such that another's must change" (Maturana, 1987, quoted in Wright & Levac, 1992). The authors concluded that "nurses are not change agents: they cannot and do not change anyone." (Wright & Levac, 1992, p. 915). The domination effects of pathologizing language set up dualities or binaries such as compliance and noncompliance. These binaries reinforce the reduced status of the patient. If nurses believed that nursing diagnoses were acts of violence against patients, Wright and Levac hold that the discipline would eliminate the language of pathologizing, called the "language of loathing" by Szaz (1973, quoted in Wright & Levac, 1992).

Nursing diagnosis also perpetuates the domination of nurse over patient by its assumption of what it means to be a person. Diagnosing from the biomedical approach becomes diagnosing defects in personhood. Such defects occur with respect to some predefined norm that the patient is not living up to—a defect in coping, self-esteem, adaptation, knowledge, and so on that nurses judge based on a superior position as social agents due to education, professional status, and power (Diers, 1986). The ideology of nursing diagnosis constitutes individuals for themselves and others in a manner that supports domination by social agents through confession and normalization of behavior in accordance with predetermined disciplinary norms. The assumption is that the individual is the source of both the problem and the solution. The responsibility for cure rests wholly on the patient in question; that is, if the patient does exactly what the nurse prescribes, the cure will be effected. On the other hand, if the patient does not perform correctly, the nurse has no responsibility for the failure to cure. Instead, the patient is given the diagnosis of noncompliance in addition to the original diagnosis. Individuals are thus constituted as targets, victims, and predictable systems to be manipulated by social agents for their own good.

For example, Carpenito (1993) claimed that many people in the United States are grieving but are not being treated because their nurse cannot identify the grief. Presumably, from a diagnosis model, these nurses are unable to recognize grief because they have not been taught what grief looks like. This talk disregards the personal knowledge of the patient and the nurse. Nurses indeed work with patients experiencing grief, but the discourse that describes "diagnosing" grief brings with it an assumption of power in a clinical encounter. The notion of "diagnosing and treating" grief is demeaning to the person who is grieving, especially when that person is told that she or he is not progressing "normally."

This mystification of common everyday concepts that already exist in the social domain of patients and nurses results in perpetuation of the domination of nurse over patient. Carpenito (1993) argues that asking a student to differentiate between anxiety and powerlessness or grieving is difficult. This argument assumes that nursing students do not already have some idea of what these words mean. The students are, in effect, being asked to deny all their previous notions of the social meaning of these terms in favor of the normalized truth from the discourse of nursing diagnosis. Then the students are instructed to apply this discourse to patients without regard to the patient's understanding of these same terms.

The concept of guilt is another example of mystification. In the discourse of nursing diagnosis, the nursing definition, interpretation, and application of concepts like guilt and grief are assumed to be appropriate because of the education and social status that goes into professional judgment and not because the nurse understands the situated individual in question. The meanings can become so generalized as to become meaningless, oppressive, and trivial. " . . . when we deal with the experiences of illness or disease, stress or joy, imprecise labeling understates the majesty of the phenomenon and the work in attending to it" (Diers, 1986, p. 30).

Grief and guilt can certainly be subjects of informed inquiry, but a method of inquiry that is based on empirical analytic foundational science necessarily promotes control strategies from power/knowledge and elitism in the application to human beings. The discourse of nursing diagnosis assumes the value of this form of inquiry only for the professional goals of elevated social status and power. Consequently, the patient is given a diagnosis that defines guilt differently from the patient's own definition, and treatment follows a standardized care plan to remedy this defect, deficit, or abnormality. When the outcome criteria are met, the diagnosis is "resolved," and the patient's power is reduced while the nurse's power is increased.

According to Kritek, "in a service discipline our clients depend on our scientific commitment to discover what is best for them" (1985, p. 6). Diagnosing defects in personhood provides the model for the highly powerful phrase, *discover what is best for them*. "Once we isolate phenomena, we can describe them, manipulate them, and create preferred outcomes; then we can have the effect we wish to have" (Kritek, 1985, p. 6). This places nurses in a social position of authority over patients viewed as targets of our power/knowledge that causes preferred outcomes. This view assumes that nurses are justified in deriving goals and interventions without full participation of patients (Allen, 1987b, p. 46). This power strategy produces uncritical clientele who are emotionally and economically dependent (Mitchell, 1991; Street, 1992).

Dickson (1993) suggested that the discourse of nursing diagnosis, informed by professionalism, implies the acceptance of a standardized, authoritarian, technical role with patients. This emphasis on control-based strategies provides the basis for the diagnosis of noncompliance. This NANDA diagnosis will be considered in some detail.

Wuest (1993b) analyzed the concept of compliance in nursing literature. She argued that the concept of compliance necessarily contains the idea of the powerful nurse and the powerless patient, but it is clothed in scientific language that disallows value critique. It follows that there is a dichotomy of compliance and noncompliance, with one valued over the other (Wright & Levac, 1992). The task of identifying and treating the condition obscures the conflict over the value of the treatment with which the patient chooses not to comply.

The justification for this domination is the professional model of social agency that is consistent with the repressive hypothesis (Powers, 1999). Diagnosing and treating noncompliance involves the patient confessing her or his intentions to the social agent, the nurse, who applies coercive treatments to normalize the patient's behavior, producing compliance as the outcome. Both the nurse and the patient assume that application of this power/knowledge is liberating instead of controlling. Calling noncompliance a diagnosis is, in effect, naming a patient decision a defect. Treating social and personal defects is the task of social agents.

Domination by Race and Culture

Domination of non-Whites by Whites and domination of cultures other than the White U.S. subculture is perpetuated by the discourse of nursing diagnosis. Geissler (1992) has supported this claim by examining three nursing diagnoses with cultural etiologies: (1) impaired verbal communication related to cultural differences, (2) impaired social interaction related to sociocultural dissonance, and (3) noncompliance related to a patient value system.

Geissler found that none of the defining characteristics meet NANDA's criteria for a major or a minor defining characteristic. By collapsing categories, seven became acceptable as minor defining characteristics. Geissler stated that "the inadequacy of the current official nursing diagnoses . . . reflects the inability to respond to cultural needs of patients" (p. 303). Geissler concluded that the "existing NANDA defining characteristics address pathophysiological causes of the inability to speak, which are irrelevant within the context of cultural/language variance" (p. 305).

Respondents to Geissler's survey objected to the use of the word *impaired*, suggesting instead that social dysfunction is culturally defined, not scientifically defined.

> The original NANDA-related factors are so broad that it would be close to impossible to plan care around them . . . The suggestions from which

the defining characteristic of ineffective communication evolved can be perceived as a problem ethnocentrically located within the nurse, not the patient. (Geissler, 1992, pp. 306–307)

Coler and her colleagues (1991) also identified problems with translating nursing diagnoses for use in Brazil, due to cultural differences from the research base of North American culture. "The NANDA diagnostic classificatory {sic} system needs to be reevaluated, reconsidered and refocused into transculturally relevant, meaningful, and useful transcultural perspectives" (Leininger, 1990, p. 24).

In 1991, Wake, Fehring, and Fadden performed what they called a "multinational search for defining characteristics of nursing diagnoses" (p. 57). They included France, Belgium, England, the United States, Canada, and Columbia. Even with this severely restricted sample, there were no common defining characteristics for hopelessness, for example. The common characteristics for anxiety were panic and nervousness. For ineffective airway clearance, the only common defining characteristic was dyspnea. The authors concluded that one of the limitations of their study was the diagnostic expertise of the nurses chosen to identify the defining characteristics. They also concluded that "Anxiety is a common human response. Manifestations of the response, however, may be influenced by culture" (p. 63).

Domination based on racial markers is also perpetuated by the language of the discourse of nursing diagnosis. Nursing students are taught specific stereotypical views of groups of people distinguished by biological markers like skin color. Nursing students are taught that stereotyping African Americans, Asian Americans, Mexican Americans and Native Americans for the purposes of individualizing "our" treatment of "them" constitutes culturally sensitive nursing care (Allman, 1992; Powers, 1992b).

The use of stereotypical views serves to perpetuate social domination of some groups by others. Race, like gender, is better conceived of as a verb, not a noun, for it is a thing we do in social situations and is not an "essential" property of reified entities. This view is nowhere represented in the essentializing discourse of nursing diagnosis.

The use of nursing diagnoses phrased in terms of "potential for (something)" is a good example of an entry point for ethnocentrism. The stereotype of the "violent Black male" can result in a diagnosis of potential aggression more often for Black male patients than for White male patients. Fernando reinforced this observation by stating that "moral characteristics, such as antisocial behavior, may be converted into (pseudo)symptoms as in the diagnostic category of psychopathy used in Western psychiatry" (1988, p. 63). Patients of color have had whole constellations of behaviors identified, diagnosed, and equated with the their non-whiteness (p. 63).

Domination based on culture and race is perpetuated by the discourse of nursing diagnosis through the process of normalization. Nursing diagnosis is a normalizing discourse that functions to bring about power effects (determined, in this case, by empirical markers) based on scientifically based knowledge assumed to be value-neutral.

Oppression of Women

The oppression of women is perpetuated by the language of the discourse of nursing diagnosis. For example, it has been demonstrated that women are more often diagnosed as manipulative or depressed than men (Allen, Allman, & Powers, 1991). This research then produces a "risk factor" in women for depression and shows up in diagnostic schemes for psychology and nursing. In a similar manner as racially identified characteristics, the risk factor is assumed to exist in the non-maleness of the patient, to be discovered and treated by the nurse, and to result in changes in the patient.

The gaze of the doctor is assumed to be that of the objective scientist (male), and the gaze of the nurse is assumed to be personal and intimate (female) (Street, 1992). The discourse of nursing diagnosis, however, is based on the male-gendered medical professional model of objective science. Thus, the personal and intimate are unacknowledged within the discourse of nursing diagnosis; the personal and intimate are devalued both in the nurse and the patient. Understanding the effect of a male-gendered professional ideology on the discourse of nursing diagnosis explains the resistance of some female nurses to using the language of the nursing diagnosis in their practice. The language is variously said to be obscure (Webb, 1992) or "pompous if not downright silly" (Curry, 1991, p. 124).

Research on diagnoses that are not oriented to context-dependent situations (Allen et al., 1991) result in descriptions of behaviors that are defined as "naturally male" or "naturally female" and therefore subsequently valued or devalued (Tannen, 1990). "The ideology of professionalism incorporates dissimulation, reification, materialism, and patriarchy in such a way as to distort reality so that it appears as 'normal' and 'natural' " (Turkoski, 1992, p. 152). In the discourse of nursing diagnosis, behaviors are not discussed as discursive subject positions that someone can choose or not choose but are discussed as "the way women are." Diagnoses categorize the constellations of feminine experience into normalizing notions that are value-laden. Women diagnosed with "ineffective coping, individual" or "impaired role performance" by a nurse would seek treatment, not seek to critique the research that generated the diagnosis.

Further research on these diagnoses in the empirical analytic tradition could result in more criteria for the nursing diagnosis of sexual role dysfunction because the woman being diagnosed does not fulfill the expectations that have been identified with being female. Both the female nurse and the female patient are thus caught up in normalized patriarchal descriptions of their own behavior and interaction.

Class Domination

Class domination is perpetuated by the discourse of nursing diagnosis. Following O'Neill, classism is defined as (1) stereotyping on the basis of economic class with resulting discrimination and (2) valuing class-based models, goals, and strategies from the dominant culture over those groups peripheralized in the society (O'Neill, 1992, p. 140).

One unintended consequence of educational elitism in nursing is that it creates tensions in people who are not from White, middle-class and owning-class backgrounds (Carnegie, 1991). The process of education within the value-laden system of nursing diagnosis results in adherence to a professional ideology that places the culture of the professional nurse in the social position of service to lower classes (Rodgers, 1991). There is no mention in the discourse of nursing diagnosis that nurses work shifts, punch time clocks, or belong to unions. This situation devalues the experience of marginalized groups in western culture.

The use of nursing diagnoses is classist in that it reinforces the assumed value of the capitalistic base of American economy. Nowhere is it mentioned in the literature on nursing diagnosis that the etiology of any of these diagnoses might be an unfair and oppressive economic system. The goal of nursing diagnosis and treatment is for the patient to adapt to current role expectations, not to change them. Not being able or willing to adapt is grounds for being given another diagnosis, most often some type of "dysfunction" or "noncompliance due to lack of knowledge" or "denial."

As an example of the assumed value of the capitalism, consider the nursing diagnosis of powerlessness, and its application to people who are homeless and jobless. Is the situation of powerlessness an alteration of some normal state of affairs to which everyone has a right? Consequently, is the intervention to get them a job or a home? To support a revolution that puts the means of production in the hands of the working class? Acknowledgment of oppressive relations in American economy is absent. Instead, the definition of *powerlessness* is "the perception that one's action will not significantly affect an outcome: a perceived lack of control over a certain situation or immediate happening" (McFarland & McFarlane, 1993, p. 505). The interventions include the following: provide opportunities for the patient to express feelings about self and illness, engage the patient in decision making whenever possible (for example, the selection of a roommate or wearing apparel), encourage a sense of partnership with the health care team, reinforce the patient's right to ask questions, teach self-monitoring, provide relevant learning materials, explore reality perceptions and clarify if necessary by providing information or correcting misinformation, and help the patient communicate effectively with other health team members (McFarland & McFarlane, 1993, p. 508).

Clearly, these strategies are control-based, giving only trivial and illusory choices and feedback to patients. When the powerlessness of the patient is related to economic circumstances, these interventions further trivialize the concerns of homeless and jobless people, ignoring the economic inequalities and perpetuating the oppression of people who are homeless and jobless.

The overwhelming emphasis of the nursing interventions in the NANDA literature involves adaptation of the patient to current circumstances, including economic circumstances, no matter how intolerable. If nurses do not always advocate adaptation to extreme circumstances with particular patients, it is reflective not of the flexibility of the taxonomy or its science, but of the overriding compassion of the individual nurse.

The official outcome criteria for the diagnosis of powerlessness are that (1) the patient verbalizes feelings of being in control of situations and outcomes, (2) the patient demonstrates adequate role functioning and coping skills, and (3) the patient exhibits appropriate mood (McFarland & Wasli, 1986). Again, in the case of the economically disadvantaged, these outcomes are demeaning and oppressive. The role of social agent thus includes assistance in developing appropriate mood and role functioning within an oppressive economic system as a given, uninterpreted reality.

Domination of Nursing by Medicine

The domination of nursing by medicine is reinforced by the discourse of nursing diagnosis because the discourse is based on the medical model of professional scientific hierarchy that is assumed to be "natural" and "normal." Nurses appropriate "both the forms of knowledge [of medicine] and the paradigm in which this knowledge is created" (Street, 1992, p. 8). It has been suggested that the choice of the word *diagnosis* is based on our paternalistic power relationship with medicine because the word *diagnosis* both separates nursing from medicine while at the same time defining nursing in the image of medicine (Kobert & Folan, 1990; Mitchell, 1991).

Thus, the discourse of nursing diagnosis reinforces the handmaiden status of nurses (Todd, 1991) by adherence to the model of the dominant group. Roberts naively asserted that using nursing diagnosis and nursing DRGs would promote more collaboration between nurses and doctors because doctors would then attend nursing diagnosis rounds (1990, p. 55). However, in 1993, there was significantly less collaboration between doctors and nurses than existed in the 1800s (Pillitteri & Ackerman, 1993). By denying the historically complex and intimate nature of the structural and social power/knowledge relations between medicine and nursing, the discourse of nursing diagnosis perpetuates the domination of nursing by medicine.

Domination of Practitioners by Academics

The discourse of nursing diagnosis also perpetuates the domination of academics over practicing nurses. Achieving professional status for nursing historically has been viewed as a more appropriate goal than that of control over the allocation of nursing knowledge and skills (O'Neill, 1992). The discourse of nursing diagnosis removes the control of practice from the individual nurses to the academic sphere.

At the fifth conference, practicing nurses were asked to respond to the conceptual framework for the classification of nursing diagnosis developed by the nurse theorists. The responses ranged from acknowledgment of potential to rejection (Kim & Moritz, 1982, pp. 264–272). The most common comments from the practicing nurses cited the time involved in documenting the nursing diagnoses using the conceptual framework, and the poorly-defined nature of "unitary man."

Goals common to all nurses have thus been separated into professional goals and working conditions. Working conditions are thereby conceived of as having little relationship to the taxonomy of nursing diagnoses. This creates a split between academics and practicing nurses. An ideology supported by the elite of nursing has the potential to split the profession into confrontational groups (Gamer, 1979).

The tension between the ideologies of education and practice can be seen within practicing nurses in the manner in which they approach the discourse of nursing diagnosis. Thompson (1985), for example, noted that practicing nurses frequently apply empiricist texts paradoxically; that is, they may approach the task of diagnosing with the preunderstanding of working class women but may also apply the taxonomy with the prejudice of aspiring intellectual professionals. The practice ideology structures the time/space of the clinical encounter in terms of the industrial, bureaucratic model.

The discourse of nursing diagnosis structures the clinical encounter in terms of the professional medical science model. "So long as nursing practice is explained as originating from, and elaborating upon, formalized theory and technological advances, bedside nurses have not had, or perhaps did not want, any particular share in it" (Maeve, 1993, p. 6). Thomas and Newsome added that "Nursing diagnosis has been a part of some nursing curricula since the '70's, but a gap still exists between theory and practice" (1992, p. 183). Turkoski noted that "there was scant evidence of nursing research directed at validating specific nursing diagnoses or the effects nursing diagnosis had on actual client care" (1988, p. 144).

Carpenito (1993), who has been involved in nursing diagnosis since 1975, identifies two kinds of opponents to nursing diagnosis: one kind of opponent who did not know anything about it and was not willing to try, and the other type who simply thought it was unnecessary jargon and just more work. Carpenito admits that practicing nurses are still reluctant to use nursing diagnosis but argues that the answer to the difficulty of using nursing diagnosis is more research.

On the other hand, Schilder and Edwards (1993) argue that it is inappropriate for academics to shift the burden of the application of research findings to practicing nurses and remedy their reluctance by educational courses. It is unlikely that more research, more in-services, or more educational instillation of ideological perspectives will remedy this reluctance (see also Wiebe, 1991).

One difficulty that practicing nurses have with nursing diagnosis is that the discourse values the general over the specific and the standard over the individual. Dickoff and James, in their 1986 commentary on their 1971 article, reflected on their idea of situation-producing theory as the way to bridge what they saw as the widening gap between academics and practicing nurses. They recognized only two choices: Practice could be based on a body of knowledge derived from situation-producing theory (such as nursing diagnosis), or practice could be left to the whim of the moment.

Dickoff and James (1989) addressed the eighth national conference with respect to academic and practicing nurses. They identified three "recoveries" necessary for the nursing diagnosis "movement," and they asked specifically, "Who has controlling say in the nursing diagnosis movement—practitioners or academicians?" (p. 101). They recommend returning control to the practitioners because, "It is not clear that the users—in the very role as users—are regarded also as developers and creators of concepts" (p. 101). One part of the "recovery" of the movement of nursing diagnosis is thus phrased by these authors in terms of the practicing nurse, not the provision of more research by academics.

Domination of Nursing in the Health Care System

The appropriate professional goal for nursing within the health care environment according to the discourse of nursing diagnosis is power and status equal to that of medicine. Using the language of the discourse of nursing diagnosis, Harrington asserts that the "ultimate goal of nursing diagnosis is to achieve adaptation [of nursing to its environment]" (Harrington, 1988, p. 94). The environment of nursing is not considered, therefore, to be changeable. The task is for nursing, using nursing diagnosis, to adapt itself to the health care environment as it exists. Carlson and her colleagues (1982) hold that "Any obstacle placed in the way of the continued development and classification of nursing diagnoses endangers the profession itself" (1982, p. 16). "Politically, nursing diagnosis has done more to advance professional practice than any other previous scientific, professional, or educational movement" (Fitzpatrick, 1990, p. 102). Woolley (1990) insisted that nursing diagnosis is the most important development for the advancement of nursing.

According to Thompson (1992), nursing in the 1970s and 1980s constructed representations of health, nursing, people, and environments. These constructions were achieved by privileged White nurses in order to secure their own location in health care dominated by business and medicine without addressing power issues. Value-less imitation of discursive practices of groups that dominate the health care system were believed to promote autonomy, independence, and the right to self-governance. However, if this can be done, then "how have respiratory therapists, physical therapists, dieticians, and paramedics, all members of professions younger than nursing, escaped this painful word searching and surged ahead to higher salaries and unquestioned professional status?" (Curry, 1991, p. 124). "Physicians have suffered no identity crises in gradually relinquishing 'medical' tasks to nurses over the years" (p. 126). The evidence for the continued oppression of nursing is ignored in the discourse of nursing diagnosis.

The "care vs. cure" debate was part of a larger movement that included the nursing diagnosis movement. The emphasis on care sought to totally dissociate nursing from its relationship to medicine, and nursing reference to the concept of disease became a serious mistake. What was called the "regressive medical paradigm" (Kritek, 1985) made treatment of disease an action that nurses disdained but imitated. Ignoring the power issues and embracing the strategy of an "end run" around the relationship with medicine perpetuates the domination of nursing in the health care system by refusing to acknowledge the issues. Participants are prevented from using anything medical in the language of nursing diagnosis by the prevailing opinion, and it was "an intensely political enterprise" (Kritek, 1985, p. 5). According to Meleis, "nor is there evidence that they [nursing diagnoses] have contributed to clarifying the nursing mission or to improving communication among nurses and with the rest of the health care team" (1991, p. 161).

The medical model of professionalism for nursing diagnosis is the most self-defeating of any possible strategy of autonomy within the health care system because of the unacknowledged assumptions of elitism based on value-less science (Street, 1992).

> To the degree that we emulate the medical model, we are tempted to believe that the development of adequate classification systems unique to the practice of nursing will differentiate us from other health professionals, assure our recognition as scientists in our own right, aid us in achieving a high level of practice, and further other goals important not only to the individual nurse but to the nursing profession as a discipline. (Douglas & Murphy, 1990, p. 17)

Later in the same article, Douglas and Murphy warn that "the nursing profession is pinning too much hope on nursing diagnosis" and "it has elevated expectations beyond a realistic level" (1990, p. 20).

RESISTANCE PRACTICES

Resistance to the oppression perpetuated by the discourse of nursing diagnosis may arise in singular instances of nursing practice involving nurses and patients or in larger group contexts. The resistance of a nurse in a hospital situation will be different from the resistance of a student, different from the resistance of a patient, and different from the resistance of an academic.

In order to identify practices of resistance to power/knowledge and to differentiate them from practices that support power/knowledge, it is helpful to ask, "Who benefits from this discourse?" Analysis of practices of resistance also has been called critical scholarship, which is defined by Thompson as "a pattern of thought and action that challenges institutionalized power relations or relations of domination in the social reality of nursing" (1987, p. 28).

The discourses of resistance acknowledged here represent potential constructed subjectivities that might resist the oppressive power effects of the discourse of nursing diagnosis in specific situations. These discourses are not discourses of resistance in and of themselves but may provide resistance subjectivities in individual situations. Co-optation of practices of resistance into the dominant discourse of nursing diagnosis will also be demonstrated.

Co-optation, like oppression, is not a consciously determined strategy of power relations. The process of incorporating minority views into a dominant discourse is viewed, in the scientific ideology, as part of the evolution of truth. To the discourse analyst this process supports the expanding influence of power/knowledge via the repressive hypothesis. Street (1992) identifies practice resistance that takes various forms, such as manipulation, passive resistance, and open critique of domination. Because the practice of nursing is an oral culture, there is a biculturalism in the discipline. Writing things down is too slow for the way a shift proceeds. Verbal report is where the crucial information is obtained and passed on to other nurses, sometimes in the form of gossip (Laing, 1993), a very devalued form of talk identified in a pejorative way with women. Written work is required, however, by medical records systems and is often performed only when the shift is over.

Nursing diagnosis is a part of the written culture of nursing viewed by some practicing nurses as being forced on practicing nurses by academics (Mitchell, 1991). The resistance activities that arise from the ideology of nursing practice, for example, take the passive form of "not doing the paperwork," or at least doing it in a perfunctory manner, because it is not easy to tell if the nurse is organizing patient care using nursing diagnosis. The academic culture of nursing interprets such passive resistance as nurses not being prepared to be held accountable for their actions and decisions (Carpenito, 1993).

Academics and administrators sometimes assume that written culture is superior to oral. They see the limitations of the oral culture for the systematic analysis of nursing practice at an abstract level (Street, 1992). "Formal explicit statements fix meaning and do not allow for nuances of interpretation the way tacit understanding does" (Gordon, 1984, p. 246). Without institutional "encouragement," it is uncommon for practicing nurses to use nursing diagnoses at all (Thomas & Newsome, 1992).

Nurse administrators have expressed the opinion that computerized nursing diagnosis provides a rich source of management data (Mehmert, Dickel, & McKeighen, 1989). The practicing nurses, on the other hand, do not value systematic analysis at the abstract level, despite what they are taught in nursing education. Their resistance is passive and unorganized (Street, 1992, p. 269).

The practices of resistance to nursing diagnosis that arise from the oral culture of nursing include an emphasis and a valuing of the intersubjective meanings of oral communication between people and the effects of communication, sharing, supporting, nurturing, interacting, learning, and teaching. Consciousness raising groups can help nurses value their own oral culture, critique power relations, and develop strategies to compile and learn from the stories of others. Street (1992) argued that nurses may become empowered to transformative, resistive action. The discourse of expertise in specific, contextualized clinical situations provides a speaking position and the words for nurses to use to express resistance to the nursing diagnosis movement.

Official co-optation of practice issues that could be developed as a source of resistance strategies is also exemplified by the concept of axes. At the ninth conference, it was suggested that axes be identified to the diagnoses in Taxonomy II (Carroll-Johnson, 1991). The justification for this is provided by Hoskins and her colleagues, who argued that the nursing community has challenged the ability of nursing diagnosis to account for nursing practice. The issues raised have become the axes, and the axes "describe the dimensions of the human condition" (1992, p. 117).

The use of axes in the system of nursing diagnosis represents an attempt to co-opt discursive practices of resistance into the dominant model, forming a classifiable entity that provides both generalized knowledge and clinical specificity. The result is tension within the discourse and overall support for expanding the controlling strategies of foundational science by co-opting the emphasis on individuality from the oral discourse of nursing practice.

Feminist discourse is a strong candidate for provision of alternative speaking positions and words that can be used to form discursive practices of resistance to the domination effects of nursing diagnosis. Nursing devalues feminist discourse in general (Dickson, 1993), and nursing diagnosis in particular avoids feminist discourse. McFarland and McFarlane (1993), for example, do not mention the word *feminist* at all. None of the research on nursing diagnosis presented in the national conferences refers to feminism.

In following the medical model of profession, White middle-class nursing leaders traditionally have severed their ties with women's groups and have allied themselves with professional groups instead. The ANA rejected a resolution supporting women's right to vote in 1908 on the grounds that it was unprofessional to have any opinion on such matters. This position was reversed in 1915, just before the passage of the Nineteenth Amendment. O'Neill says the ANA's stand on the Equal Rights Amendment (ERA) was even worse, and the NLN never publicly supported the ERA (O'Neill, 1992, p. 143).

According to Street (1992), the discourse of nursing diagnosis reflects a desire to emulate the oppressor, which Street names as medicine. She calls nursing diagnosis an example of liberal feminism, where the focus is on equal rights within the same oppressive system, without a focus on changing the system itself, by limiting participation to White, middle class, heterosexual females (p. 52). Feminist critique of nursing diagnosis would serve to point out the gendered nature and sexist consequences of the discourse (DeMarco,

Campbell, J., & Wuest, J., 1993). The use of the language of postmodern feminism would provide the words to deconstruct the power relations inherent in the use of the discourse of nursing diagnosis.

Postmodern feminist discourse that addresses power relations and feminist research practices that include such strategies as consciousness-raising groups have potential for providing position descriptions and action strategies to critique the power relations of nursing diagnosis. Furthermore, postmodern feminist discourse is less likely to be co-opted into the discourse of nursing diagnosis than, for example, caring or expert practice discourse. This is due to the assumption of the preferability of the postmodern approach to knowledge generation as opposed to the androcentric scientific professional model.

The Discourse of Ethical Practical Morality as Resistance

Ethical discussions are devalued in a discourse that assumes a foundational perspective because the entire body of knowledge is assumed to be value-free in both its construction and application. On the other hand, Maeve believed, citing Bishop and Scudder (1991), that the dominant sense of nursing in general is moral and personal, as opposed to professional and technical (1993, p. 10). Levine claimed that all nursing actions have a moral component (1989). The marginalized discourse of ethics and practical morality in nursing literature argues that this approach could give nursing authority (Dickson, 1993). These discourses could provide ways of talking and acting that could be used by individual practitioners, academics, and administrators to resist the oppressive power relations of nursing diagnosis.

As an example of providing a way of talking that resists oppressive power relations, consider Mitchell's (1991) ethical analysis of nursing diagnosis. Mitchell claimed that human suffering is created by the diagnostic process in nursing diagnosis (p. 99). She argued that being forced to use nursing diagnoses puts nurses in ethical conflicts (p. 102) and causes unacknowledged stress, suffering, and tension in their practice. Much more effort in the approach of ethical analysis could be supported in order to provide more examples of ethical dilemmas in nursing practice. Such an approach does not ignore the power relations inherent in nursing practice.

Patient Advocacy as Resistance

The discourse of patient advocacy is related to the practical, moral perspective and can also give rise to ideological subjectivities that provide practices of resistance to the oppressive power relations of nursing diagnosis. Porter (1992) argued that the attempt by nursing to achieve social agency by the attainment of a body of nursing knowledge such as nursing diagnosis contradicts the role of advocacy for nurses. He argued specifically that this oppressive situation further devalues the voice of patients and their families because they are considered the targets of the intervention, not as sources of knowledge.

To be a patient advocate is to mediate between the patient and a more powerful social system. Nursing diagnosis places nursing more solidly within the powerful social system and further away from patient situations and perspectives, making advocacy more difficult. Although nurses do advocate for patients, more often they advocate for doctors to patients, because they share the same commitment to the medicalization of increasing portions of life.

As a source of strategies of resistance, advocacy provides words and actions that can be used to structure alternative nursing actions. Nursing has a moral and practical basis for moving beyond the hospital setting to advocate on a global basis concerning issues such as hunger, violence, homelessness, AIDS, poverty, children's rights, and primary health care (Dickson, 1993, p. 81). Nursing could encourage a talent for putting information into terms patients can understand (Curry, 1991) and could provide support for decisions that might be unpopular with the health care system in general or could even be inconsistent with the nurse's own viewpoint, by admitting the voice of patients into the clinical encounter.

Union Discourse as Resistance

The discourse of unionism as a source of talk about power is devalued by the discourse of nursing diagnosis because it is not viewed as part of the professional, scientific ideology. Antiunionism appeals to the classism in nursing and separates nurses from a possible source of resistance strategies (Allen, 1987a). In following the medical model of a profession, White middle-class nursing leaders removed the links with women's groups and unions and allied themselves with male professional groups, isolating themselves from alliances that could provide models of strength that are not male- or science-based (Allen, 1987). There is no union language in the discourse of nursing diagnosis and no discussion that the work of the majority of nurses is "shift work."

The use of union discourse and strategies has potential to form a speaking position to resist oppressive power relations related to nursing diagnosis because union talk already acknowledges class-based oppression. Nurses who acknowledge class-based oppression would be more likely to acknowledge instances of class-based oppression as a result of the application of the discourse of nursing diagnosis. The discourse of unionism is a promising source of alternative ideologies to the professionalizing influence of nursing diagnosis on the clinical encounter. The vision of nursing as a pink collar occupation can provide for practices that resist the oppressive effects of nursing diagnosis on patients in the clinical encounter.

Empowerment and Social Action as Potential Resistance Discourses

Roberts (1983), Hedin (1986), Skillings (1992), and Ricci (1993) all argued that nurses are an oppressed group and describe examples of behavior that demonstrate this, such as horizontal violence and cultures of silence. Because nursing is female-gendered, it has a long history of oppression. Citing Reverby (1987), for example, Ricci (1993) observed that the models of hierarchy, responsibility, and discipline that were used to shape American nursing were adapted not only from the Victorian family but also from the military.

Since nurses function as an oppressed group, the skills used by nurses to resist what they consider to be oppressive both within and without nursing do not reflect open critique of domination. The binary conceptualizations that are constructed include the mental versus the manual and the written versus the oral. Nurses feel oppressed by forces outside of nursing, such as medicine, and by academics and management nurses within the discipline. Nursing diagnosis is considered another oppressive condition within the practice of nursing. The skills of resistance included in the repertoire of an oppressed group are largely passive and indirect. Therefore, nurses resist the discourse of nursing diagnosis with silence, foot dragging, and complaining.

Using the discourse of empowerment as a source of alternative speaking positions would provide nursing with strategies, processes, and words to resist individual practices of domination from nursing diagnosis as they arose. The concept of empowerment means people coming into a recognition of their own power (Lather, 1991). Empowerment is not a strategy that one person or group uses on another person or group. One person cannot empower another; the direction of action arises from within. Speaking a language of empowerment, nurses might organize consciousness raising groups in the workplace in order to provide group resistance to nursing diagnosis in that setting. Speaking a language of empowerment, individual nurses might justify their work with patients without using the language of nursing diagnosis.

The discourse of empowered social activism that could arise from this potential source of resistance is easily co-opted by nursing diagnosis, however. Consider the following diagnosis that is supposed to be treated by nursing: "Altered Health Maintenance related to inability to secure adequate permanent housing for self and family" (McFarland & McFarlane, 1993, p. 23). One of the symptoms of this condition is "verbalization of inaccurate information." The political, economic, and power aspects of this patient situation are ignored. Expressing inaccurate information is a "symptom" of altered health maintenance. Any possible discourse concerning social action aimed at provision of adequate housing is diverted into assessment of the ability of the patient to tell the truth.

Talk of empowerment can thus be easily co-opted to refer to a "task" for a social agent, instead of a "process" by which some person or group comes to knowledge of their own power in resistance to social agency. When co-opted, it becomes the task of nursing to "empower" patients or researchers to "empower" research subjects or educators to "empower" students (Mason, Becker, & Georges, 1991; Parker & McFarlane, 1991.) In this "empowerment as a treatment" model, patients are considered "empowered" when they are no longer noncompliant with treatments and when they make choices that the nurse, as a social agent, considers wise. In the case of nursing diagnosis, "empowerment" of nurses is seen by the proponents of nursing diagnosis as supported when nurses use the discourse in practice (Carpenito, 1993). The definition of empowerment as given previously, however, implies that empowered nurses might choose not to use the discourse of nursing diagnosis.

Empowerment is a complex discourse. Public health nurses have been identified as performing both empowering and coercive strategies within the same case, often being unable to untangle the concepts used in the intervention (Zerwekh, 1992). As a potential source of strategies for resisting oppression, however, empowerment could be widely supported with further writing and discussion.

The Voice of the Patient as Resistance

The voice of the patient was found to be completely absent from the discourse of nursing diagnosis. Patients are constituted according to the discourse as the targets of the interventions, not as participants in the discourse. Individual differences between patients are treated by the discourse as research variables, amenable to standardization. Patients are not invited to conferences or invited to submit diagnoses for consideration. Panels of patients are not given diagnoses to review. Patients are not acknowledged to have any appropriate place in the discourse at all. They are the objects of the gaze of the discourse; they do not participate in the gaze.

The voice of the patient could be solicited within the discourse or could be viewed as a subjectivity with potential to articulate resistance to the oppressive effects of nursing diagnosis within the clinical encounter. This position might be difficult to solicit since many patients believe the repressive hypothesis and accept their oppressed position in the clinical encounter, especially when they have been defined as "not healthy." The grid of power relations in the clinical encounter is more complicated than simply that of nurse over patient. In other words, the voice of the patient is difficult to find but necessary to hear.

The power relations within which the discourse of nursing diagnosis functions are complex. Turkoski argued that the female emulation of a male professional ideology that includes racism, sexism, and classism has the unintended consequences of denigration of our own members as females, causing horizontal violence and hierarchical pressures within the occupation with respect to education, race, class, and gender. Understanding the ideology as male-gendered makes sense of such situations as the ANA's rejection of women's issues outside the occupation in favor of alliances with other (male) professions.

CONCLUSIONS

The concluding claims of this discourse analysis are as follows.

1. There is evidence that the discourse of nursing diagnosis depends on, reproduces, and extends conditions of social domination. The discourse uses notions of science, normality, and the role of social agency, which constitute individuals for themselves and others in an oppressive manner according to hierarchical categories. These categories are determined by empirical markers such as race, gender, and class, limiting autonomy and responsibility in a systematic manner but not by purposeful design.

2. There is evidence that the discourse of nursing diagnosis restricts what counts as evidence and limits acceptable input of voices into the structure and functioning of the clinical encounter to those social agents with scientific nursing expertise, thus excluding, for example, the voice of the patient and the patient's family.

3. The discourse of nursing diagnosis suppresses discussion relating to the operation of power and resistance to power by appeal to the dominance of empirical analytic science with foundational assumptions and equates this dominance with professional social status. This results in the perpetuation of oppressed group behavior among practicing nurses by creating tensions within the practice of nursing between competing discourses as potential subjective speaking positions.

The models available at the time of the development of nursing diagnosis were limited to male- and power-based constructions that now conflict with other traditions in nursing thought. Based on an assumption of value-free power/knowledge, nursing diagnosis has widespread influence and serious consequences in the United States. Evidence for these claims has been provided. Potential discourses of resistance that provide speaking positions from which to articulate specific practices that resist oppressive effects of nursing diagnosis have also been provided.

Discourse analysis can be considered an important approach in nursing inquiry because some of the problematic notions that underlie the various discourses within nursing are not, strictly speaking, empirically based. Instead, the notions are conceptual and discursive, concerned with assumptions and power relations. "Discursive analyses of texts are not simply descriptions or analyses of content: rather, they are critical and reflexive, moving beyond the level of common sense" (Cheek, 2000, p. 42). "Discourse analysis is both interpretive and explanatory" (Titscher, Meyer, Wodak & Vetter, 2000, p. 146).

The marginalized discourses of empowerment and social action, feminism, a wider view of scientific activity and knowledge, advocacy, and power can be given more exposure and can be recognized as valid perspectives for nursing. These perspectives help to emphasize, for example, the process by which the subject matter for inquiry is illuminated, instead of focusing entirely on the subject matter itself. Nursing could also contribute to the academy by utilizing contemporary developments in the approach to analysis and demonstrating what revised conceptualizations of research and scholarship could mean in a practice discipline.

Wuest (1993a) points out that the traditional method of concept analysis in nursing, in seeking the universal critical attributes of a concept, loses the elements that reveal androcentric bias. The nature of the relationship and character of the decision-making process fail to emerge (p. 7). "One cannot rehabilitate lives in a social structure that is directed to their dehumanization" (Lichtman, 1982, p. 284).

Canguilhem (1978) emphasized that normal and abnormal are not descriptive terms; rather, they are evaluative terms. Health and illness are not opposites or even ends of a continuum. "To be in good health means being able to fall sick and recover, it is a biological luxury" (p. 7). We must consider it normal for the pathological to occur. Canguilhem argued that what is statistically frequent is not necessarily normal, and what is statistically infrequent is not necessarily abnormal and surely not pathological. A revised notion of normal, combined with an emphasis on an individual clinical situation and consideration of the inherent power relations, is a promising approach to the generation of nursing knowledge. This approach can be considered both scholarly and rigorous.

The intentions of the original proponents of nursing diagnosis were timely and well thought out, but the models available then were limited. The unintended consequences are now being played out. The discourse of nursing diagnosis constitutes a discourse phrased in modern professional scientific terms and based on an exclusionary and elitist model of power. The influence that the discourse seeks in its description of the clinical encounter for the purpose of determining truth within that sphere does not impinge upon the turf of medicine, because if it did, nursing would now be facing powerful opposition or co-optation. The sphere of influence we are carving out comes instead from patients and their families, and we are using the language of science, professionalism, and medicine to justify ignoring these voices.

As stated by Gordon, "Nursing, in trying to differentiate nursing expertise, to move beyond obedience to medical orders, and to become more autonomous and accountable can ill afford to reinforce impersonality and mere obedience by adding more rules that tend to restrict judgment" (1984, p. 232).

BIBLIOGRAPHY

Abdellah, F. (1957). Methods of identifying covert aspects of nursing problems. *Nursing Research*, 6(1), 4–23.

Abdellah, F. (1969). The nature of nursing service. *Nursing Research*, 18, 390–393.

Adamson, P. B. (1991). Symptoms in ancient mesopotamia. *Medical History*, 35(4).

Alexander, J. (1992). General theory in the postpositivist mode: The 'epistemological dilemma' and the search for present reason. In S. Seidman & D. Wagner (Eds.), *Postmodernism and social theory*. Cambridge, MA: Blackwell.

Allen, D. (1985). Nursing research and social control: Alternative models of science that emphasize understanding and emancipation. *Image*, 17, 58–64.

Allen, D. (1986). Using philosophical and historical methodologies to understand the concept of health. In P. Chinn (Ed.), *Nursing research methodology: Issues and implementations* (pp. 157–168). Rockville, MD: Aspen Systems.

Allen, D. (1987a). Professionalism, occupational segregation by gender, and control of nursing. *Women and Politics*, 6(3), 1–24.

Allen, D. (1987b). The social policy statement: A reappraisal. *Advances in Nursing Science*, 10(1), 39–48.

Allen, D., Allman, K., & Powers, P. (1991). Feminist research without gender. *Advances in Nursing Science*, 13(3), 49–58.

Allen, D., Benner, P., & Diekelman, N. (1986). Three paradigms for nursing research: methodological implications. In P. Chinn (Ed.), *Nursing Research Methodology: Issues and Implementations*. Rockville, MD: Aspen Systems.

Allen, D. G. (1986). The use of philosophical and historical methodologies to understand the concept of health. In P. Chinn (Ed.), *Nursing research methodology: Issues and implementations*. Rockville, MD: Aspen Systems.

Allen, D. G. (1991). Applying critical social theory to nursing education. In N. Greenleaf (Ed.), *Curriculum revolution: Redefining the student-teacher relationship*. New York: NLN.

Allen, D. G. (1992). Feminism, relativism, and the philosophy of science: An overview. In J. L. Thompson, D. G. Allen, & L. Rodrigues-Fisher (Eds.), *Critique, resistance, and action: Working papers in the politics of nursing*. New York: NLN.

Allman, K. M. (1991). Theories of the body: Situated knowledges and critical narratives. In D. G. Allen, K. M. Allman, & P. Powers (Eds.), *Taken-For-Grantedness in Nursing* (Monograph). Australia: Deakin University.

Allman, K. M. (1992). Race, racism, and health: Examining the 'natural' facts. In J. L. Thompson, D. G. Allen, & L. Rodrigues-Fisher (Eds.), *Critique, resistance, and action: Working papers in the politics of nursing*. New York: NLN.

Althusser, L. (1971). Ideology and ideological state apparatuses. In *Lenin and Philosophy*. New York: Modern Reader.

American Association of Critical Care Nurses. (1990). *Outcome standards for nursing care of the critically ill*. Laguna Niguel, CA: author.

American Nurses Association. (1973). *Standards of nursing practice*. Kansas City, MO: author.

American Nurses Association. (1980). *Nursing: A social policy statement*. Kansas City, MO: author.

American Nurses Association. (1989). *Classification systems for describing nursing practice*. Kansas City, MO: author.

American Nurses Association. (1991). *Standards of clinical nursing practice*, Kansas City, MO: author.

American Nurses Association. (1995). *Letter from V.T. Betts to E. O'Neill*. Washington, DC: author.

Anderson, J. E., & Briggs, L. L. (1988). Nursing diagnosis: A study of quality and supportive evidence. *Image*, 20(3), 141–144.

Anderson, L. K. (1991). Orientation based on nursing diagnosis. Old concepts in today's practice. *AORN*, 54(4), 826–830.

Aronowitz, S. (1992). The tensions of critical theory: Is negative dialectics all there is? In S. Seidman, & D. Wagner (Eds.), *Postmodernism and social theory*. Cambridge, MA: Blackwell.

Aspinal, M. J. (1976). Nursing diagnosis: The weakest link. *Nursing Outlook*, 24, 433–437.

Avant, K. C. (1990). The art and science in nursing diagnosis development. *Nursing Diagnosis*, 1(2), 51–56.

Baker, C. (1993). The advocacy paradigm: You want big stories, don't you? Paper presented at the 4th annual conference on Critical and Feminist Perspectives in Nursing, Atlanta, GA.

Barnum, B. J. (1990). On nursing. *Nursing and Health Care*, 11(5), 227.

Benner, P. (1990). Response to hermeneutic inquiry. In L. Moody, *Advancing Nursing Science Through Research, Volume Two*. Newbury Park, CA: Sage.

Benner, P. (1984). *From novice to expert: Excellence and power in clinical nursing practice*. Menlo Park, CA: Addison-Wesley.

Bernauer, J., & Rasmussen, D. (Eds.). (1988). *The final Foucault*. Cambridge: MIT Press.

Bernstein, R. (1986). *Beyond objectivism and relativism*. Philadelphia: University of Penn. Press.

Bevis, E., & Watson, J. (1989). *Toward a caring curriculum: A new pedagogy for nursing*. New York: NLN.

Beyea, S. C. (1990). Concept analysis of feeling: A human response pattern. *Nursing Diagnosis*, 1(3), 97–101.

Bircher, A. U. (1986). Nursing diagnosis: Where does the conceptual framework fit? In M. E. Hurley (Ed.), *Classification of Nursing Diagnoses: Proceedings of the Sixth Conference* (pp. 66–104). St. Louis, MO: Mosby.

Bishop, A., & Scudder, J. (1991). *Nursing: The practice of caring*. New York: NLN.

Bond, M. E. (1988). Knowledge deficit: Not a nursing diagnosis. *Image*, 20(3), 141–144.

Booth, B. (1992). Nursing diagnosis: One step forward. *Nursing Times*, 88(7), 32–33.

Boyer, E. (1990). *Scholarship reconsidered: Priorities for the professoriate*. Princeton, NJ: The Carnegie Foundation for the Advancement of Teaching.

Brown, R. H. (1992). Social science and society as discourse: Toward a sociology for civic competence. In S. Seidman, & D. Wagner (Eds.), *Postmodernism and social theory*. Cambridge, MA: Blackwell.

Bulechek, G. M. (1987). Promotion of nursing diagnoses through state nurses association. *Nursing Clinics of North America*, 22(4), 1002–1009.

Bulechek, G. M., Kraus, V. L., Wakefield, B.,& Kowalski, D. K. (1990). An evaluation guide to assist with implementation of nursing diagnosis. *Nursing Diagnosis*, 1(1), 18–23.

Bulechek, G. M., & McCloskey, J. C. (1990). Nursing intervention taxonomy development. In J. McCloskey, & H. Grace, *Current issues in nursing*, (3rd ed., pp. 23–28). St. Louis, MO: Mosby.

Burns, C. (1991). Development and content validity testing of a comprehensive classification of diagnoses for pediatric nurse practitioners. *Nursing Diagnosis*, 2, 95–103.

Byers, J. (1988). *From Hippocrates to Virchow*. Chicago: ASCP Press.

Bynum, W. F., & Nutton, V. (Eds.) (1981). *Theories of fever from antiquity to enlightenment, medical history supplement #1*. London: Welcome Institute.

Calhoun, C. (1992). Culture, history and the problem of specificity in social theory. In S. Seidman, & D. Wagner (Eds.), *Postmodernism and social theory*. Cambridge, MA: Blackwell.

Campbell, J., & Bunting, S. (1991). Voices and paradigms: Perspectives on critical and feminist theory in nursing. *Advances in Nursing Science*, 13(3), 1–15.

Canguilhem, G. (1978). *On the normal and the pathological*. Dordrecht, Holland: Reidel.

Carlson, J., Craft, C., & McGuire, A. (Eds.) (1982). *Nursing diagnosis*. Philadelphia: Saunders.

Carnegie, M. E. (1991). *The path we tread: Blacks in nursing 1854–1990* (3rd ed.). New York: NLN.

Carpenito, L. (1989). Developments in nursing classification. In *American Nurses Association classification systems for describing nursing practice* (pp. 13–19). Kansas City, MO: ANA.

Carpenito, L. (1993, April). Speaking the language of nursing diagnosis. *Critical Care Nurse*, 91–97.

Carpenito, L. (1995). *Nursing diagnosis: Application to clinical practice*, (6th ed.). Philadelphia: Lippincott.

Carroll-Johnson, R. M. (1989). *Classification of nursing diagnoses: Proceedings of the eighth conference*. Philadelphia: Lippincott.

Carroll-Johnson, R. M. (1991). *Classification of nursing diagnoses: Proceedings of the ninth conference*. Philadelphia: Lippincott.

Chambers, W. (1962). Nursing diagnosis. AJN, 62(11), 102–104.

Cheek, J. (2000). *Postmodern and Poststructural Approaches to Nursing Research*. Thousand Oaks, CA: Sage.

Chinn, P. (1985). Debunking myths in nursing theory and research. *Image*, 17(2), 45–49.

Chinn, P. L., & Jacobs M. K. (1978). A model of theory development in nursing. *Advances in Nursing Science*, 1(1), 1–11.

Clark, J., & Lang, N. (1992). Nursing's next advance: An international classification for nursing practice. *International Nursing Review*, 39(4), 109.

Clinton, J. (1986). Nursing diagnoses research methodologies. In M. E. Hurley (Ed.), *Classification of nursing diagnoses: Proceedings of the sixth conference* (pp. 159–167). St. Louis, MO: Mosby.

Clunn, P. (1984). Nurses' assessment of a person's potential for violence: Use of grounded theory in developing a nursing diagnosis. In M. J. Kim, et al., *Classification of nursing diagnosis: Proceedings of the fifth national conference* (pp. 376–393). St. Louis, MO: Mosby.

Coler, M. S., Lima da Nobrega, M. M., de Almeida Peres, V. L., & Nunes de Farias, J. (1991). A Brasilian study of two diagnoses in the NANDA human response pattern, moving: A transcultural comparison. In R. M. Carroll-Johnson, *Classification of nursing diagnoses: Proceedings of the ninth conference* (pp. 255–256). Philadelphia: Lippincott.

Condon, E. H. (1992). Nursing and the caring metaphor: Gender and the political influences on an ethic of care. In J. L. Thompson, D. Allen, & L. Rodrigues-Fisher, *Critique, resistance and action: Working papers in the politics of nursing* (pp. 69–83). New York: NLN.

Creason, N. S. (1992, June). How useful are urinary incontinence nursing diagnoses? Urologic Nursing, 46–47.

Curry, J. (1991). Nursing diagnosis: Communication, impaired. Journal of Emergency Nursing, 17(3), 124–126.

Curtin, L. (1978). The nurse as advocate: A philosophical foundation for nursing. Advances in Nursing Science, 1 (3), 1–10.

DeMarco, R., Campbell, J., & Wuest, J. (1993). Feminist critique: Searching for meaning in research. Advances in Nursing Science, 16(2), 26–38.

Dennison, P. D., & Keeling, A. W. (1989). Clinical support for eliminating the nursing diagnosis of knowledge deficit. Image, 21(3), 142–144.

Derdiarian, A. (1988). A valid profession needs valid diagnoses. Nursing and Health Care, 9(3), 137–140.

Diamond, I., & Quinby, L. (1988). Feminism and Foucault: Reflections on resistance. Boston: Northeastern University Press.

Dickoff, J., & James, P. (1986). Commentary. In L. Nicoll, Perspectives on Nursing Theory. Boston: Little, Brown and Company.

Dickoff, J., James, P., & Wiedenbach, E. (1968). Theory in a practice discipline, Part I: Practice oriented theory. Nursing Research, 17(5).

Dickson, G. L. (1990). A feminist poststructuralist analysis of the knowledge of menopause. Advances in Nursing Science, 12(3), 15–31.

Dickson, G. L. (1993). The unintended consequences of a male professional ideology for the development of nursing education. Advances in Nursing Science, 15(3), 67–83.

Diers, D. (1986). On Words. Image, 18(2), 30.

Doering, L. (1992). Power and knowledge in nursing: A feminist poststructuralist view. Advances in Nursing Science, 14(4), 24–33.

Donaldson, S. K., & Crowley, D. (1978). The discipline of nursing. Nursing Outlook, 26(2), 113–120.

Douglas, D. J., & Murphy, E. K. (1990). Nursing process, nursing diagnosis, and emerging taxonomies. In J. McCloskey & H. Grace, Current Issues in Nursing (3rd ed.). St. Louis, MO: Mosby.

Dreyfus, H., & Rabinow, P. (1983). Michel Foucault, beyond structuralism and hermeneutics. Chicago: University of Chicago Press.

Dreyfus, H. (1987). Foucault's critique of psychiatric medicine. Journal of Medicine and Philosophy, 12(4), 311–333.

Dreyfus, H., & Rabinow, P. (1983). Michel Foucault: Beyond structuralism and hermeneutics (2nd ed.). Chicago: University of Chicago Press.

Durand, M. & Prince, R. (1966). Missing diagnosis: process and decision. Nursing Forum, 5, 51–64.

Dzurec, L. (1989). The necessity for and evolution of multiple paradigms for nursing research: A poststructuralist perspective. Advances in Nursing Science, 11(4), 69–77.

Edel, M. (1982). The nature of nursing diagnosis. In J. Carlson, C. Craft, & A. McGuire (Eds.), Nursing Diagnosis (pp. 3–17). Philadelphia: Saunders.

Eldridge, I., & Levi, M. (1982). Collective bargaining as a power resource for professional goals. Nursing Administration Quarterly, 6(2), 29–40.

Ellis, R. (1983). Philosophical inquiry. *Annual Review of Nursing Research*, 1, 211–228.

England, M. (1989). Nursing diagnosis: A conceptual framework. In Fitzpatrick and Whall, *Conceptual Models of Nursing*, (2nd ed., pp. 347–369). Englewood Cliffs, NJ: Appleton and Lange.

Estes, J. W. (1989). *The medical skills of ancient Egypt*. Canton, MA: Science History Publications.

Fawcett, J. (1986). Guest editorial: Conceptual models of nursing, nursing diagnosis, and nursing theory development. *Western Journal of Nursing Research*, 8(4), 397–399.

Fawcett, J. (1990). Comment on a unified nursing diagnositic model. *Image*, 22(4), 263.

Fehring, R. J. (1986). Validating diagnostic labels: Standardized methodology. In M. E. Hurley (Ed.), *Classification of nursing diagnoses: Proceedings of the sixth conference*. St. Louis, MO: Mosby.

Fernando, S. (1988). *Race and culture in psychiatry*. New York: Routledge.

Fitzpatrick, J. J. (1987). Etiology: Conceptual concerns. In A. M. McLane, *Classification of nursing diagnoses: Proceedings of the seventh conference* (pp. 61–64). St. Louis: Mosby.

Fitzpatrick, J. J. (1990). Conceptual basis for the organization and advancement of nursing knowledge: Nursing diagnosis/taxonomy. *Nursing Diagnosis*, 1(3), 102–106.

Fitzpatrick, J. J. (1991). Taxonomy II: Definitions and development. In R. M. Carroll-Johnson, *Classification of nursing diagnoses: Proceedings of the ninth conference* (pp. 23–29). Philadelphia: Lippincott.

Fitzpatrick, J. J., Kerr, M. E., Saba, V. K., Hoskins, L. M., Hurley, M. E., Mills, W. C., Rottkamp, B. C., Warren, J. J., & Carpenito, L. J. (1989). Translating nursing diagnosis into ICD code. *American Journal of Nursing*, 89, 493–495.

Fleishman, E. A. (1982). Systems for describing human tasks. *American Psychologist*, 37, 821–834.

Forsyth, G. L. (1984). Etiology: In what sense and of what value? In M. J. Kim, G. K. McFarland, & A. M. McLane (Eds.), *Classification of nursing diagnoses: Proceedings of the fifth national conference* (pp. 63–72). St. Louis, MO: Mosby.

Foss, S. K., & Gill, A. (1987). Michel Foucault's theory of rhetoric as epistemic. *Western Journal of Speech Communication*, 51, 384–401.

Foucault, M. (1965). *Madness and civilization* (R. Howard, Trans.). New York: Vintage/Random House.

Foucault, M. (1970). *The order of things*. New York: Vintage/Random House.

Foucault, M. (1972). *The archaeology of knowledge and the discourse on language* (A. M. Sheridan-Smith, Trans.). New York: Pantheon.

Foucault, M. (1975). *The birth of the Clinic* (A. M. Sheridan-Smith, Trans.). New York: Vintage/Random House.

Foucault, M. (1979). *Discipline and Punish: the Birth of the Prison*, translated by Alan Sheridan. New York: Vintage/Random House.

Foucault, M. (1979). *Discipline and punish: The birth of the prison*, (A. Sheridan, Trans.). New York: Vintage/Random House.

Foucault, M. (1978, 1985, 1986). *The History of Sexuality, Volumes 1, 2, and 3* (R. Hurley, Trans.). New York: Random House.

Foucault, M. (1988). The political technology of individuals. In Martin, Gutman, & Hutton (Eds.), *Technologies of the self*. Amherst: University of Massachusetts Press.

Foucault, M. (1977). *Knowledge, counter-memory, and practice: Selected essays and interviews* (D. F. Bouchard, Ed.). Ithaca, NY: Cornell Press.

Frank, B. (1990). Back to basics. *Journal of Professional Nursing, 6,* 326.

Fraser, N. (1989). *Unruly practices: Power, discourse and gender in contemporary social theory.* Minneapolis: University of Minnesota Press.

Fredette, S. L. (1988). Common diagnostic errors. *Nurse Educator, 13*(3), 31–35.

Friedson, E. (1970). Profession of Medicine— A study of the sociology of applied knowledge. New York: Dodd Mead.

Friere, P. (1971). *Pedagogy of the oppressed.* New York: Continuum.

Fry, V. (1953). The creative approach to nursing. AJN, 53(3), 301–302.

Galdston, I. (1981). *Social and historical foundations of modern medicine.* New York: Brunner-Mazel.

Gamer, M. (1979, February). The ideology of professionalism. *Nursing Outlook,* 108–111.

Gavey, N. (1989). Feminist poststructuralism and discourse analysis. *Psychology of Women Quarterly, 13,* 459–475.

Gebbie, K. (Ed.) (1976). *Classification of nursing diagnoses: Summary of the second national conference.* St. Louis, MO: Clearinghouse-National Group for Classification of Nursing Diagnosis.

Gebbie, K. (1989). Major classification systems in health care and their use. In American Nurses Association, *Classification Systems for Describing Nursing Practice* (pp. 48–49). Kansas City, MO: ANA.

Gebbie, K., & Lavin, M. (1975). *Classification of nursing diagnoses: Proceedings of the first national conference.* St. Louis, MO: Mosby.

Gebbie, K. M. (1982). Towards the theory development for nursing diagnosis classification (1978). In M. J. Kim & D. A. Moritz, *Classification of nursing diagnoses: Proceedings of the third and fourth national conferences* (pp. 8–14). New York: McGraw-Hill.

Geissler, E. M. (1992). Nursing diagnoses: A study of cultural relevance. *Journal of Professional Nursing, 8*(5), 301–307.

Giddens, A. (1987). *Social theory and modern sociology.* Stanford, CA: Stanford University Press.

Gordon, D. R. (1984). Research application: Identifying the use and misuse of formal models in nursing practice. In P. Benner, *From novice to expert: Excellence and power in clinical nursing practice.* Menlo Park, CA: Addison-Wesley.

Gordon, M. (1976). Nursing diagnosis and the diagnostic process. AJN, 76, 1276–1300.

Gordon, M. (1982a). *Nursing diagnosis: Process and application.* New York: McGraw-Hill.

Gordon, M. (1982b). Guidelines for nursing diagnosis development and workshops. In M. J. Kim & D. A. Moritz, *Classification of nursing diagnoses: Proceedings of the third and fourth national conferences* (pp. 339–341). New York: McGraw-Hill.

Gordon, M. (1987). *Nursing diagnosis: Process and application* (2nd ed.). New York: McGraw-Hill.

Gordon, M. (1990). Toward theory-based diagnostic categories. *Nursing Diagnosis, 1*(1), 5–11.

Gray, D. P. (1992). A feminist critique of Jean Watson's theory of caring. In J. L. Thompson, D. Allen, & L. Rodrigues-Fisher, *Critique, resistance and action: Working papers in the politics of nursing* (pp. 85–96). New York: NLN.

Griffith, M. (1989). Historical perspective and ANA policies. In *American Nurses Association classification systems for describing nursing practice* (pp. 4–5). Kansas City, MO: ANA.

Grmek, M. D. (1989). *Diseases in the ancient Greek world.* Baltimore, MD: Johns Hopkins University Press.

Gross, E., & Pateman, C. (1986). *Feminist challenges: Social and political theory.* Sydney: Allen & Unwin.

Habermas, J. (1971). *Knowledge and human interests.* Boston: Beacon Press.

Habermas, J. (1984). *The theory of communicative action, vol. 1 and 2.* Boston: Beacon Press.

Hagey, R. S., & McDonough, P. (1984). The problem of professional labeling. *Nursing Outlook, 32,* 151–157.

Hall, L. (1955). Quality of nursing care. *New Jersey State Department of Health, Public Health News, 36,* 212–213.

Hall, J. M., & Stevens, P. E. (1995) The Future of graduate education in nursing: Scholarship, the health of communities, and health care reform. *Journal of Professional Nursing, 11*(6), 332–338.

Hall J. M., Stevens, P. E., & Meleis, A. I. (1994) Marginalization: A guiding concept for valuing diversity in nursing knowledge. *Advances in Nursing Science, 16*(4), 23–41.

Harrington, L. W. (1988). The diagnosis dilemma: One preferred remedy. *Nursing and Health Care, 9*(2), 92–94.

Harvey, R. M. (1993). Nursing diagnosis by computers: An application of neural networks. *Nursing Diagnosis, 4*(1), 26–34.

Hedin, B. A. (1986). A case study of oppressed group behavior in nurses. *Image, 18*(2), 53–57.

Heinrich, K. T., & Witt, B. (1993). The passionate connection: Feminism invigorates the teaching of nursing. *Nursing Outlook, 41,* 117–124.

Hekman, S. (1986). *Hermeneutics and the sociology of knowledge.* Notre Dame: University of Notre Dame Press.

Held, D. (1980). *Introduction to critical theory: Horkheimer to Habermas.* Berekley: University of California Press.

Henderson, B. (1978). Nursing diagnosis: Theory and practice. *Advances in Nursing Science, 1*(1), 75–83.

Henderson, V. (1994). *Virginia Henderson the nurse theorists: Portraits of excellence* [Videotape]. Oakland, CA: The Helene Fuld Health Trust.

Hiraki, A. (1992). Language and the reification of nursing care. In J. L. Thompson, D. Allen, & L. Rodrigues-Fisher, *Critique, resistance and action: Working papers in the politics of nursing.* New York: NLN.

Hirsch, M., & Chang, B. L. (1990). Collaboration for the development of a nursing diagnosis system. *Western Journal of Nursing Research, 12*(5), 693–697.

Hornung, G. J. (1956). The nursing diagnosis—an exercise in judgement. *Nursing Outlook, 4*(1), 29–30.

Hoskins, L. M., Fitzpatrick, J. J., Warren, J. J., Avant, K., Carpenito, L. J., Hurley, M. E., Jakof, D., Lunney, M., Mills, W. C., & Rottkamp, B. C. (1992). Axes: Focus of Taxonomy II. *Nursing Diagnosis*, 3(3), 117–123.

Hudson, R. P. (1983). *Disease and its control: The shaping of modern thought.* Westport, CT: Greenwood Press.

Hutchinson, S. (1987). Police story. *Image*, 19(3), 153.

Iowa Intervention Project.(1992). *Nursing interventions classification* (NIC). St. Louis, MO: Mosby.

Iowa Intervention Project. (1993a). The NIC Taxonomy Structure. *Image*, 25(3), 187–192.

Iowa Intervention Project. (1993b) NIC *interventions linked to* NANDA *diagnoses.* Iowa City: University of Iowa Press.

Jacobs, K., & Huether, S. (1978). Nursing science: The theory-practice linkage. *Advances in Nursing Science*, 1(1), 63–73.

Jacox, A. (1974). Theory construction in nursing: An overview. *Nursing Research*, 23, 4.

Jenny, J. (1987). Knowledge deficit: Not a nursing diagnosis. *Image*, 19(4), 184–185.

Joint Commission on Accreditation of Healthcare Organizations. (1992). *Accreditation manual for hospitals.* Oakbrook Terrace, IL: author.

Joint Commission on Accreditation of Healthcare Organizations. (1995). *Accreditation manual for hospitals.* Oakbrook Terrace, IL: author.

Kalisch, P., & Kalisch, B. (1995). T*he advance of American nursing* (3rd ed.) Philidelphia: Lippincott.

Keeling, A., Utz, S. W., Shusler, G. F., & Boyle, A. (1993). Non-compliance revisited: A disciplinary perspective of a nursing diagnosis. *Nursing Diagnosis*, 4(3), 91–97.

Kerr, M. E. (1991). Validation of taxonomy. In R. M. Carroll-Johnson, *Classification of nursing diagnoses: Proceedings of the ninth conference* (pp. 6–13). Philadelphia: Lippincott.

Kikuchi, J. F., & Simmons, H. (1992). *Philosophical inquiry in nursing.* Newbury Park, CA: Sage.

Kim, H. S. (1983). *The nature of theoretical thinking in nursing.* Norwalk, CN: Appleton-Century-Crofts.

Kim, M. J., McFarland, G. K., & McLane, A. M. (Eds.). (1984). *Classification of nursing diagnosis: Proceedings of the fifth national conference.* St. Louis, MO: Mosby.

Kim, M., & Moritz, D. (1982). *Classification of nursing diagnoses: Proceedings of the third and fourth national conferences.* New York: McGraw-Hill.

King, L. S. (1967). What is a diagnosis? Journal of the American Medical Association, 202 (8), 714–717.

Kirsch; E. (1991). Treating nursing's response to nursing diagnosis. Journal of *Emergency Nursing*, 17(3) 125–126.

Kobert, L., & Folan, M. (1990). Coming of age in nursing: Rethinking the philosophies behind holism and nursing process. *Nursing and HealthCare*, 11(6), 308–312.

Komorita, N. I. (1963). Nursing diagnosis. AJN, 63(12), 83–85.

Kritek, P. (1978). The Generation and classification of nursing diagnosis: Toward a theory of nursing. *Image*, 10(2), 33–40.

Kritek, P. (1984). Current nomenclature and classification systems: Pertinent issues. In M. J. Kim, G. K. McFarland, & A. M. McLane (Eds.), *Classification of nursing diagnoses: Proceedings of the fifth national conference* (pp. 73–88). St. Louis, MO: Mosby.

Kritek, P. B. (1985). Nursing diagnosis in perspective: response to a critique. *Image* 17 (3) p. 3–8.

Kritek, P. (1986). Development of a taxonomic structure for nursing diagnoses: A review and an update. In M. E. Hurley (Ed.), *Classification of nursing diagnoses: Proceedings of the sixth conference* (pp. 23–38). St. Louis, MO: Mosby.

Kritek, P. (1989). An introduction to the art and science of taxonomy. In American Nurses Association, *Classification systems for describing nursing practice* (pp. 6–12). Kansas City, MO: ANA.

Kuhn, T. (1970). *The structure of scientific revolutions* (2nd ed.). Chicago: University of Chicago Press.

Kusch, M. (1991). *Foucault's strata and fields: An investigation into archaeological and genealogical science studies.* Dordrecht, The Netherlands: Kluwer Academic Publishers.

Laing, M. (1993). Gossip: Does it play a role in the socialization of nurses? *Image*, 25(1), 37–43.

Lang, N. M. (1986). Classification, taxonomy, structure. In M. E. Hurley (Ed.), *Classification of nursing diagnoses: Proceedings of the sixth conference* (pp. 15–22). St. Louis, MO: Mosby.

Lang, N., Galliher, J., & Hirsch, I. (1989). Challenge to the profession. In American Nurses Association, *Classification systems for describing nursing practice* (pp. 70–73). Kansas City, MO: ANA.

Lang, N. M., & Gebbie, K. (1989). Nursing taxonomy: NANDA and ANA joint venture toward ICD-10CM. In R. M. Carroll-Johnson, *Classification of nursing diagnoses: Proceedings of the eighth conference* (pp. 11–17). St. Louis, MO: Mosby.

Lang, N., & Marek, K. (1990). The classification of patient outcomes. *Journal of Professional Nursing*, 6, 158–163.

Lather, P. (1991). *Getting smart.* New York: Routledge.

Lee, H., & Strong, K. (1985). Using nursing diagnosis to describe the clinical competence of baccalaureate and associate degree graduating students: A comparative study. *Image*, 17(3), 82–85.

Leininger, M. (1990). Issues, questions, and concerns related to the nursing diagnosis cultural movement from a transcultural nursing perspective. *Journal of Transcultural Nursing*, 2(1), 23–32.

Leonard, S. T. (1990). *Critical theory in political practice.* Princeton: Princeton University Press.

Leslie, C. (1990). Scientific racism: Reflections on peer review, science and ideology. *Social Science and Medicine*, 31(3), 891–912.

Levin, D., & Solomon, G. (1990). The discursive formation of the body. *Journal of Medicine and Philosophy*, 15, 515–537.

Levin, R. F., (1989). Diagnostic content validity of nursing diagnosis. *Image*, 21(1), 40–44.

Levine, M. E. (1966). Trophicognosis: An alternative to nursing diagnosis. *ANA's regional clinical conference: Exploring progress in medical surgical nursing.* New York: ANA.

Levine, M. E. (1987). Approaches to the development of a nursing diagnosis taxonomy. In A. M. McLane, *Classification of nursing diagnoses: Proceedings of the seventh conference* (pp. 45–52). St. Louis, MO: Mosby.

Levine, M. E. (1989). The ethics of nursing rhetoric. *Image*, 21(1), 4–6.

Lichtman, R. (1982). *The production of desire*. New York: MacMillan.

Lieb, R. (1978). Power, powerlessness, and potential: Nurses' role within the health care delivery system. *Image*, 10(3), 75–83.

Lindberg, D. C. (1991). *The beginnings of western science*. Chicago: University of Chicago Press.

Lindsay, A. M. (1990). Identification and labeling of human responses. *Journal of Professional Nursing*, 6(3), 143–50.

Logan, J., & Jenny, J. (1990). Deriving a new nursing diagnosis through qualitative research: Dysfunctional ventilatory weaning response. *Nursing Diagnosis*, 1(1), 37–43.

Loomis, M. E., O'Toole, A. W., Brown, M. S., Pothier, P., West, P., Wilson, H. S. (1987). Development of a classification system for psychiatric/mental health nursing: Individual response class. *Archives of Psychiatric Nursing*, 1(1), 16–24.

Loveridge, J. (1990). Rethinking the 'parenting' paradigm: Embodied mothers and fathers in discourse/practice. *Early Child Development and Care*, 55, 17–25.

Lowenberg, J. S. (1993). Interpretive research methodology: Broadening the dialogue. *Advances in Nursing Science*, 16(2), 57–69.

Lunney, M. (1990). Accuracy of nursing diagnoses: Concept development. *Nursing Diagnosis*, 1(1), 12–17.

Lupton, D. (1992). Discourse analysis: A new methodology for understanding the ideologies of health and illness. *Australian Journal of Public Health*, 16(2), 145–50.

Maas, M. L. (1987). Organizational characteristics that facilitate the use of nursing diagnoses. *Nursing Clinics of North America*, 22(4), 881–886.

Maas, M. L.; Hardy, M. A., & Craft, M. (1990). Some methodologic considerations in nursing diagnosis research. *Nursing Diagnosis*, 1(1), 24–30.

Maeve, M. K. (1993). The carrier bag theory of nursing practice. Paper presented at the 4th annual Critical and Feminist Perspectives in Nursing Conference, Atlanta, GA.

Marek, K. (1989). Classification of outcome measures in nursing care. In American Nurses Association, *Classification systems for describing nursing practice* (pp. 37–42). Kansas City, MO: ANA.

Martin, K. (1989). Omaha system. In American Nurses Association, *Classification systems for describing nursing practice* (pp. 43–47). Kansas City, MO: ANA.

Martin, L. H., Gutman, H., & Hutton, P. H. (1988). *Technologies of the self, a seminar with Michel Foucault*. Amherst: University of Massachusetts: Press.

Mason, D. Backer, B. A., Georges, C. A. (1991). Toward a feminist model for the empowerment of nurses. *Image*, 23(2), 72–77.

Matlock (1975). *The belief in the progress of medicine*. Unpublished thesis, University of Washington, Seattle.

Matthews, C. A. & Gaul, A. L. (1979). Nursing diagnosis from the perspective of concept attainment and critical thinking. *Advances in Nursing Science, vol. 2*, 17–26.

Maturana, H. (speaker) (1987). The Sin of Certainty (video tape). University of Calgary: Calgary, Alberta, Canada.

Mauksch, H. (1990). Has the frontline nurse been abandoned? In J. McCloskey & H. Grace, *Current issues in nursing* (pp. 484–489). St. Louis, MO: Mosby.

McCloskey, J. C. (1987). Taxonomy I letter, *Image*, 19(4), 216.

McCloskey, J. C., Bulechek, G. M., Cohen, M. Z., Craft, M. J., Crossley, J. D., Denehy, J. A., Glick, O. J., Kruckeberg, T., Maas, M., Prophet, C. M., Tripp-Reimer, T. (1990). Classification of nursing interventions. *Journal of Professional Nursing*, 6, 151–157.

McCloskey, J. C., & Bulechek, G. (1993). The NIC Taxonamic Structure: Iowas Intervention Project. *Image*, 25 (3) 187–192.

McCourt, A. (1986). Nursing diagnoses: Key to quality assurance. In M. E. Hurley (Ed.), *Classification of nursing diagnoses: Proceedings of the sixth conference* (pp. 133–142). St. Louis, MO: Mosby.

McFarland, G., & McFarlane, E. (1993). *Nursing diagnosis and intervention, planning for patient care* (2nd ed.). St. Louis, MO: Mosby.

McFarland, G., & Wasli, E. (1986). *Nursing diagnoses and process in psychiatric mental health nursing*. Philadelphia: Lippincott.

McIntosh, P. (1988). *White privilege and male privilege: A personal account of coming to see correspondences through work in women's studies* (Working Paper No. 189). Wellesley, MA: Wellesley College.

McLane, A. M. (Ed.) (1987). *Classification of nursing diagnoses: Proceedings of the seventh conference*. St. Louis, MO: Mosby.

McManus, R. L. (1951). Assumption of functions in nursing. In Teachers College, Columbia University, *Regional planning for nurses and nursing education*. New York: Columbia University.

Mehmert, P. A., Dickel, C. A., & McKeighen, R. J. (1989). Computerizing nursing diagnosis. *Nursing Management*, 20(7), 24–26, 28, 30.

Meleis, A. (1991). *Theoretical nursing: Development and progress* (2nd ed.). New York: Lippincott.

Melosh, B. (1979). *Skilled hands, cool heads, and warm hearts: Nurses and nursing, 1920–1960*. Unpublished dissertation. Providence, RI: Brown University.

Metzger, K. L., & Hiltunen, E. (1986, March). Diagnostic content validation of ten frequently reported nursing diagnoses. Paper presented at the meeting of the NANDA, St. Louis, MO.

Mish'alani, J. K. (1988). Michel Foucault and philosophy: An overview. Unpublished paper. U. of Washington, Seattle.

Mitchell, G. (1991). Nursing diagnosis: An ethical analysis. *Image*, 23(2).

Mitchell, G. J. & Santopinto, M. (1988, November). An alternative to nursing diagnosis. *Canadian Nurse*, 25–28.

Mundinger, M., & Jauron, G. (1975). Developing a nursing diagnosis. *Nursing Outlook*, 23, 94.

NANDA. (1992). NANDA *nursing diagnoses: Definitions and classification 1992–1993*. Philadelphia: author.

NANDA. (1994). NANDA news. *Nursing Diagnosis*, 5(2),:52–53.

Nietzsche, F. W. (1967). *On the genealogy of morals*. Translated by Walter Kaufman & R. J. Hollingdale, New York: Vintage Books.

Nettleton, S. (1989). Power and pain: The location of pain and fear in dentistry and the creation of a dental subject. *Social Sciences and Medicine*, 29(10), 1183–1190.

Newman, M. A. (1987). Nursing's emerging paradigm: The diagnosis of pattern. In A. M. McLane, *Classification of nursing diagnoses: Proceedings of the seventh conference* (pp. 53–60). St. Louis, MO: Mosby.

Nicholson, L. (1992). On the postmodern barricades: Feminism, politics, and theory. In S. Seidman, & D. Wagner (Eds.), *Postmodernism and social theory*. Cambridge, MA: Blackwell.

Niziolek, C., & Shaw, S. M. (1991). Professional practice. Whose plan—whose care? *Journal of Professional Nursing*, 7(3), 145.

Nutton, V. (1983). The seeds of disease: An explanation of contagion and infection from the Greeks to the Renaissance. *Medical History*, 27, 2–34.

O'Neill, J. (1986). The medicalization of social control. *Canadian Review of Sociology and Anthropology*, 23(3), 350–364.

O'Neill, S. (1992). The drive for professionalism in nursing: A reflection of classism and racism. In J. Thompson, D. Allen, & L. Rodrigues-Fisher (Eds.), *Critique, resistance, and action: Working papers in the politics of nursing*. New York: NLN.

Oxford English Dictionary. (1989). Oxford, England: Clarendon Press.

Parker, B., & McFarlane, J. (1991). Feminist theory and nursing: An empowerment model for research. *Advances in Nursing Science*, 13(3), 59.

Parse, R. R. (1981). *Man-living-health: A theory of nursing*. New York: John Wiley.

Passmore, J. (1967). Logical positivism. In Paul Edwards (Ed.), *The encyclopedia of philosophy, volume five* (pp. 52–57). New York: Macmillan.

Phaneuf, M. C. (1985). *Issues in professional nursing practice: 7 standards of nursing practice*. Kansas City, MO: American Nurses Association.

Pillitteri, A., & Ackerman, M. (1993). The 'doctor-nurse game': A comparison of 100 years—1888–1990. *Nursing Outlook*, 41, 113–116.

Pokorny, B. E. (1985). Validating a diagnositic label: Knowledge deficit. *Nursing Clinics of North America*, 20(4), 641–655.

Popkess-Vawter, S. (1991). Wellness nursing diagnoses: To be or not to be? *Nursing Diagnosis*, 2(1), 19–25.

Porter, E. J. (1986). Critical analysis of NANDA nursing diagnosis taxonomy I. *Image*, 18(4), 136–139.

Porter, S. (1992). The poverty of professionalization: A critical analysis of strategies for the occupational advancement of nursing. *Journal of Advanced Nursing*, 17(6), 720–726.

Powers, P. (1988). *Nurse recruitment in the AJN*. Unpublished paper. University of Manitoba, Winnipeg.

Powers, P. (1992a). *The case for philosophical inquiry*. Unpublished paper. University of Washington, Seattle.

Powers, P. (1992b). *Michel Foucault's concept of power applied to nursing's concepts of individual and environment*. Unpublished paper. University of Washington, Seattle.

Powers, P. (1996). Discourse analysis as a methodology for nursing inquiry. *Nursing Inquiry*, 3(4), 207–217.

Powers, P. (1999). Applying the concept of need to patient empowerment. In H. S. Kim & I. Kollak (Eds), *Nursing theories: Conceptual and philosophical foundations*. New York: Springer.

Pridham, K. F., & Schutz, M. E. (1985). Rationale for a language for naming problems from a nursing perspective. *Image*, 17(4), 122–127.

Puterbaugh, S., Koralewski, K., & Falkenhagen, K. (1987). Nursing diagnoses challenged. AORN, 46(4), 612, 614.

Ramprogus, V. (1995) *The deconstruction of nursing*. Brookfield, VT: Avebury.

Rasch, R. F. R. (1987). The nature of taxonomy. *Image*, 19(3), 147–149.

Rawlinson, M. (1987). Foucault's strategy: Knowledge, power, and the specificity of truth. *Journal of Medicine and Philosophy*, 12(4), 372–395.

Reeder, F. (1991). Hermeneutics. In B. Sarter, *Paths to knowledge: Innovative research methods for nursing* (pp. 193–237). New York: NLN Publication No. 15-2233.

Reverby, S. (1989). *Ordered to care*. Cambridge, MA: Cambridge U. Press.

Ricci, K. (1993). Horizontal violence in nursing: Is it rooted in the educational process? Paper presented at the 4th annual Critical and Feminist Perspectives in Nursing, Atlanta, GA.

Ricour, P. (1983). *Hermeneutics and the human sciences*, (J. Thompson, Trans.) London: Cambridge University Press.

Roberts, S. J. (1983). Oppressed group behavior: Implications for nursing. *Advances in Nursing Science*, 5(7), 21–30.

Roberts, S. L. (1990). Achieving professional autonomy through nursing diagnosis and nursing DRG's. *Nursing Admin Quarterly*, 14(4), 54–60.

Rodgers, B. L. (1991). Deconstructing the dogma in nursing knowledge and practice. *Image*, 23(3), 177–181.

Rogers, M. E. (1963). Building a strong education foundation. AJN, 63, 165–177.

Rorty, R. (1979). *Philosophy and the mirror of nature*. Princeton, NJ: Princeton University Press.

Roy, C. (1975). The impact of nursing diagnosis. AORN, 21, 1023.

Roy, C. (1984). Framework for classification systems development: Progress and issues. In M. J. Kim, G. McFarland, & A. McFarlane (Eds.), *Classification of nursing diagnosis: Proceedings of the fifth national conference* (pp. 26–45). St. Louis, MO: Mosby.

Rushton, J. P., & Bogaert, A. F. (1989). Population differences in susceptibility to AIDS: An evolutionary analysis. *Social Science and Medicine*, 28(12), 1211–1220.

Saba, V. K. (1989). Nursing information systems. In American Nurses Association, *Classification systems for describing nursing practice* (pp. 55–61). Kansas City, MO: ANA.

Sarter, B. (1988). *Paths to knowledge: Innovative research methods for nursing*. New York: NLN.

Scahill, L. (1991). Nursing diagnosis vs. goal-oriented treatment planning in in-patient child psychiatry. *Image*, 23(2).

Schilder, E., & Edwards, M. (1993). Nursing research, are we headed in the right direction? Paper presented at the 4th annual Critical and Feminist Perspectives in Nursing Conference, Atlanta, GA.

Schon, D. (1983). *The reflective practitioner: How professionals think in action*. New York: Basic Books.

Schumacher, K. L., & Gortner, S. R. (1992). (Mis)conceptions and reconceptions about traditional science. *Advances in Nursing Science*, 14(4), 1–11.

Schuster, E. (1993). Greening the curriculum. *Journal of Nursing Education*, 32(8), 381–383.

Scott, C. (1987). The power of medicine, the power of ethics. *Journal of Medicine and Philosophy*, 12(4), 334–350.

Seidel, G. (1993). The competing discourses of HIV/AIDS in sub-Saharan Africa: Discourses of rights and empowerment vs. discourses of control and exclusion. *Social Sciences and Medicine*, 36(3), 175–194.

Seidman, S. (1992). Postmodern social theory as narrative with a moral intent. In S. Seidman, & D. Wagner (Eds.), *Postmodernism and social theory*. Cambridge, MA: Blackwell.

Seidman, S., & Wagner, D. (Eds.). (1992). *Postmodernism and social theory*. Cambridge, MA: Blackwell.

Shamansky, S. L. & Yanni, C. R. (1983). In opposition to nursing diagnosis: A minority opinion. *Image*, 15(2), 47–50.

Shoemaker, J. K. (1989). Nursing diagnosis in graduate curricula. *Journal of Professional Nursing*, 5(3), 140–143.

Silva, M. C., & Rothbart, D. (1984). An analysis of changing trends in philosophies of science on nursing theory development and testing. *Advances in Nursing Science*, 6(2), 1–13.

Skillings, L. N. (1992). Perceptions and feelings of nurses about horizontal violence as an expression of oppressed group behavior. In J. Thompson, D. Allen, & L. Rodrigues-Fisher (Eds.), *Critique, resistance, and action: Working papers in the politics of nursing*. New York: NLN.

Smith, M. J. (1988). Perspectives on nursing science. *Nursing Science Quarterly*, 1(2), 80–85.

Smythe, E. (1993). The teacher as midwife: A New Zealand narrative. *Journal of Nursing Education*, 32(8), 365–369.

Spicker, S. (1987). Introduction to the medical epistemology of Georges Canguilhem: Beyond Michel Foucault. *Journal of Medicine and Philosophy*, 12(4), 397–411.

Stelzer, F., & Becker, A. (1982). In J. Carlson, C. Craft, & A. McGuire (Eds.), *Nursing Diagnosis* (pp. 18–32). Philadelphia: Saunders.

Stenberg, M. J. (1979). Ethics as a component of nursing education. *Advances in Nursing Science*, 1(3), 53–61.

Stewart, J., & D'Angelo, G. (1988). *Together: Communicating interpersonally* (3rd ed). New York: Random House.

Stolte, K. M. (1996). *Wellness: Nursing diagnosis for health promotion*. Philadelphia: Lippincott.

Street, A. F. (1992). *Inside nursing, a critical ethnography of clinical nursing practice*. Albany, NY: State U. of NY Press.

Swanson, K. M. (1991). Empirical development of a middle range theory of caring. *Nursing Research*, 40, 161–166.

Swanson, K. M. (1993). Nursing as informed caring for the well-being of others. *Image*, 25(4), 352–357.

Sweeney, S. S. (1990). Traditions, transitions, and transformations of power in nursing. In J. C. McCloskey & H. K. Grace (Eds.), *Current issues in nursing* (3rd ed, pp. 459–465). St. Louis, MO: Mosby.

Szasz, T. (1973). The Second Sin. New York: Anchor Press/Doubleday.

Tannen, D. (1990). *You just don't understand: Women and men in conversation.* New York: Ballantine.

Tanner, C. (1993). Nursing education and violence against women. *Journal of Nursing Education,* 32(8), 339–340.

Tavris, C. (1982). *Anger: The misunderstood emotion.* New York: Touchstone.

Taylor, F. K. (1979). *The concepts of illness, disease, and morbus.* Cambridge, UK: Cambridge University Press.

Thomas, N. M., & Newsome, G. G. (1992). Factors affecting the use of nursing diagnosis. *Nursing Outlook,* 40(4), 182–186.

Thompson, J. (1984). *Studies in the theory of ideology.* Berkeley: University of California Press.

Thompson, J. L. (1985). Practical discourse in nursing: Going beyond empiricism and historicism. *Advances in Nursing Science,* 7(4), 59–71.

Thompson, J. L. (1987). Critical scholarship: The critique of domination in nursing. *Advances in Nursing Science,* 10(1), 27–38.

Thompson, J. L. (1990). Hermeneutic inquiry. In L. Moody, *Advancing nursing through research, vol. 2.* Newbury Park, CA: Sage.

Thompson, J. L. (1992). Identity politics, essentialism, and constructions of 'home' in nursing. In J. L. Thompson, D. G. Allen, & L. Rodrigues-Fisher (Eds.), *Critique, resistance, and action: Working papers in the politics of nursing.* New York: NLN.

Tierney, A. (1987). Days of judgment. *Nursing Times,* 83(28), 19.

Tinkle, M., & Beaton, J. (1983). Toward a new view of science: Implications for nursing research. *Advances in Nursing Science,* 5, 17–36.

Titscher, S., Meyer, M., Wodak, R. & Vetter, E. (2000). *Methods of Text and Discourse Analysis.* Thousand Oaks, CA: Sage.

Todd, F. (1991). Guest editorial on nursing diagnosis applauded. *Journal of Emergency Nursing,* 17(6), 365–366.

Toth, R. M. (1984). Reimbursement mechanism based on nursing diagnosis. In M. J. Kim, G. K. McFarland, & A. M. McLane (Eds.), *Classification of nursing diagnoses: Proceedings of the fifth national conference,* (pp. 90–102). St. Louis, MO: Mosby.

Turkoski, B. (1988). Nursing diagnosis in print, 1950–1985. *Nursing Outlook,* 36(3) 142–144.

Turkoski, B. (1992). A critical analysis of professionalism in nursing. In J. L. Thompson, D. G. Allen, & L. Rodrigues-Fisher (Eds.), *Critique, resistance, and action: Working papers in the politics of nursing* (pp. 149–165). New York: NLN.

van Dijk, T. A. (1987). *Communicating racism: Ethnic prejudice in thought and talk.* Newbury Park, CA: Sage.

Vincent, K., & Coler, M. (1990). A unified nursing diagnostic model. *Image,* 22(2), 93–95.

Visitainer, M. A. (1986). The nature of knowledge and theory in nursing. *Image,* 18(2), 32–38.

Wake, M. M., Fehring, R. J., & Fadden, T. (1991). Multi-national validation of anxiety, hopelessness and ineffective airway clearance. *Nursing Diagnosis,* 2(2), 57–64.

Walker, L., & Avant, K. (1988). *Strategies for theory construction in nursing* (2nd ed.). San Mateo, CA: Appleton and Lange.

Watson, J. (1985). *Nursing: Human science and human care.* Norwalk, CT: Appleton-Century-Crofts.

Watson, J. (1990). Caring knowledge and informed moral passion. *Advances in Nursing Science,* 13(2), 15–24.

Webb, C. (1992). Nursing diagnosis: Or two steps back. *Nursing Times,* 88(7), 33–34.

Webster, G. (1984). Nomenclature and classification system development. In M. J. Kim, G. K. McFarland, and A. M. McLane (Eds.), *Classification of nursing diagnoses: Proceedings of the fifth national conference* (pp. 14–25). St. Louis, MO: Mosby.

Weedon, C. (1987). *Feminist practice and poststructuralist theory.* Oxford: Blackwell.

Werley, H. H., & Zorn, C. R. (1989). The nursing minimum data set and its relationship to classifications for nursing practice. In American Nurses Association, *Classification systems for describing nursing practice* (pp. 50–54). Kansas City, MO: ANA.

Wiebe, D. (1991). More applause for guest editorial on nursing diagnosis. *Journal of Emergency Nursing,* 17(6), 366.

Wilson, J. V. K., & Reynolds, E. H. (1990). Translation and analysis of a cunieiform text forming a part of a Babylonian treatise on epilepsy. *Medical History,* 34, 185–198.

Wooldridge, J. B., Brown, O. F., & Herman, J. (1993). Nursing diagnosis: The central theme in nursing knowledge. *Nursing Diagnosis,* 4(2), 50–55.

Wooley, N. (1990). Nursing diagnosis: Exploring the factors which may influence the reasoning process. *Journal of Advanced Nursing,* 15(1), 110–117.

Wright, L. M., & Levac, A. M. C. (1992). The non-existence of non-compliant families: The influence of Humberto Maturana. *Journal of Advanced Nursing,* 17, 913–917.

Wuest, J. (1993a). *Concept analysis: A feminist approach.* Paper presented at the 4th annual Critical and Feminist Perspectives in Nursing Conference, Atlanta, GA.

Wuest, J. (1993b). Removing the shackles: A feminist critique of non-compliance. *Nursing Outlook,* 41, 217–224.

Yamato, G. (1990). Something about the subject makes it hard to name. In G. Anzaldua (Ed.), *Making face, making soul haciendo caras.* San Francisco: Aunt Lute Foundation.

Yarling, R., & McElmurry, B. (1986). The moral foundation of nursing. *Advances in Nursing Science,* 3(2), 63–73.

Yura, H., & Walsh, M. (1973). *The nursing process: Assessing, planning, implementing, evaluating* (2nd ed.). New York: Appleton-Century-Crofts.

Zerwekh, J. (1992). The practice of empowerment and coercion by expert public health nurses. *Image,* 24(2), 101–105.

AUTHOR INDEX